Tropical Diseases

including aspects of hygiene, malnutrition and injuries

Sister Christine Hoverd

N.S.S.J.D., R.G.N., R.M., M.T.D.

Rosemary Brown

B.Sc. (Hons), R.G.N., R.M., H.V. Cert, C.T.C.M. and H.

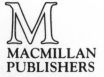

MACMILLAN
PUBLISHERS

First published 1986

Published by *Macmillan Publishers Ltd*
London and Basingstoke
Associated companies and representatives in Accra,
Auckland, Delhi, Dublin, Gaborone, Hamburg, Harare,
Hong Kong, Kuala Lumpur, Lagos, Manzini, Melbourne,
Mexico City, Nairobi, New York, Singapore, Tokyo

ISBN 0-333-42346-1

Printed in Hong Kong

British Library Cataloguing in Publication Data
Hoverd, Christine
  Tropical diseases: including aspects
  of hygiene, malnutrition and injuries.—
  (Tropical health concise notes)
  1. Tropical medicine
  I. Title II. Brown, Rosemary III. Series
  616.9'88'3   RC961
ISBN 0-333-42346-1

Acknowledgements
The authors and publishers wish to thank the following who have kindly given permission for the
use of copyright material:—
Butterworth Scientific Ltd. for the 'Food Square' from *Paediatric Priorities in Developing Countries*
by D Morley.
Churchill Livingstone, Edinburgh, for the table 'Normal Values' from *Principles and Practice of*
Medicine by Sir Stanley Davidson 11th Edition.
Oxford University Press for the Vaccination table adapted from *Refugee Community Health Care*
edited by Simmonds, Vaughan and Gunn, and two tables from *Manual on Feeding Infants and*
Young Children by Cameron and Hofvander.
Oxford University Press for the following drawings p 16; p 17; p 18; p 49; p 55 (both); p 64; p 89
from *Primary Child Care 1: A Manual for Health Workers* by Maurice & Felicity King & Soebagio
Martodipoero (1978)
Text photographs courtesy of WHO
Front cover photograph, Larval form of dog tapeworm *Echinococcus granulosus* from hydatid cyst,
courtesy of Science Photo Library; Sinclair Stammers

Contents

Acknowledgements

We would like to express our appreciation to all those who, during our time abroad and in our tropical medicine courses, helped greatly to increase our knowledge of tropical health problems. Without them this book would not have been written.

Dedication

This book was based on a series of lectures given at the British Hospital for Mothers and Babies shortly before it closed in July 1984.

As such, we write it remembering with pride and affection all that B.H.M.B. stood for — its Christian witness, high professional standards and individualised care.

We hope these may be perpetuated elsewhere in the years to come, especially in those places where this book is used.

I would like to dedicate this book with thanks to my parents and brother who have always given me so much encouragement.

I would also like to dedicate it to all my friends in Africa and at the Liverpool School of Tropical Medicine who have taught me so much both by word and deed.

Rosemary Brown

I would like to dedicate this book to my parents and the community of the nursing sisters of St. John the Divine of which I am a member.

I would also like to dedicate it to the memory of B.H.M.B. and to students and midwives working throughout the developing world.

Christine N.S.S.J.D.

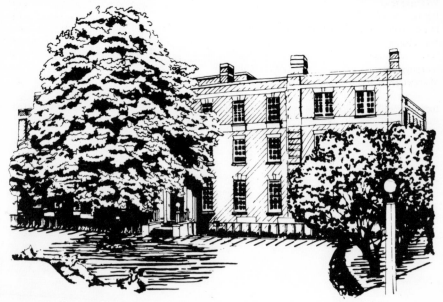

Drawing by Christopher Tucker

Preface

By now you will probably have read several books on the health problems in developing countries, and had the appropriate lectures that accompany them. This little book is not meant to replace these but to complement them and assist you in sorting out the priorities and revising each subject in a logical, concise way. We hope that it will also provide you with a useful reference tool, so that you will be able to find quickly important information you need in your practice as a health worker.

Further reading

The following books are suggested as giving the best overall information that is currently available on various aspects of health care. Space is left for you to add titles of books that you have found particularly helpful.

Bell, D. R. (1981) *Lecture Notes on Tropical Medicine* Blackwell Scientific Publications.

Cameron, M. and Hofvander, Y. (1983) *Manual on Feeding Infants and Young Children* Oxford University Press (available from TALC).

Essex, B. J. (1977) *Diagnostic Pathways in Clinical Medicine: a epidemiological approach to clinical problems* (2nd edition) Churchill Livingstone.

King, M., King, F. and Martodipoero, S. (1978) *Primary Child Care: A Manual for Health Workers, Book 1* Oxford University Press (available from TALC).

Morley, D. (1973) *Paediatric Priorities in Developing Countries* E.L.B.S. and Butterworth (available from TALC).

Werner, D. (1977) *Where There is no Doctor* Macmillan Publisher (available from TALC).

Werner, D. and Bower, B. (1982) *Helping Health Workers Learn* The Hesperian Foundation (available from TALC; excellent if you will be involved in any kind of teaching).

Introduction

What do we need to bear in mind when talking about tropical medicine?

1 Medical problems cannot be isolated from other problems
One of the biggest problems today is that of increasing populations and decreasing national resources.

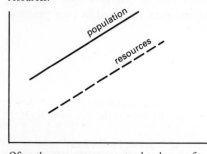

Often the resources never stand a chance of keeping up with the demands of a rising population.

Often what happens is that the resources decrease in relation to the rise in population.

Maybe resources are diverted towards cash crops rather than towards growing food for the local population.

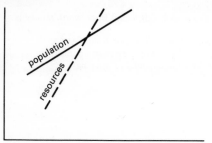

For development to take place resources need to be greater than the current demand of the population

or the rise in the population needs to be curbed to allow this to occur.

A rise in population will increase the demand on all resources including:
- food
- water
- wood or other fuel for fires
- materials for house building
- schooling
- work
- medical services
- land used for agriculture and development

Therefore, medical problems must be seen in the whole social context. Medical care helps but it is not sufficient by itself as the following chart on pages 8 and 9 shows.

2 Priorities need to be carefully thought through
First, a comprehensive survey of the situation in which you are working is vital if you are to provide the most appropriate health care. Important considerations are
- location
- climate
- soil (which affects vegetation and crops)
- insect and animal pests
- water supplies and sanitation
- communications (roads, transport, etc.)
- age/sex ratio of the population
- family and community groups
- beliefs and traditions
- education and literacy
- occupations
- housing

Next, specific questions about health should be considered:
- nutrition (What do people eat? Is it adequate?)
- common diseases
- role of traditional healers and midwives
- what health services are available locally (hospitals, vaccination, antenatal and children's clinics, etc.)

3 Local customs and beliefs of the population will affect the use of the health services
What do people in your area do when they are ill? Perhaps they
- fail to recognize the illness and what causes it
- fail to understand the severity of the illness
- ignore the illness because it is chronic or common
- believe that the illness will run its course without treatment
- deny the illness (e.g. leprosy) because of the shame attached to it

Where do people go for help? They might
- go nowhere, because of fear, ignorance or distrust of the health services, distance from health services or difference in language and culture between the patient and the person treating them
- rely on themselves, using traditional remedies or drugs obtained from dispensaries or from an unofficial source
- go to the local traditional healer
- or they may come to government-sponsored mission or private health care facilities, i.e. us!

What should be our attitude towards local customs and beliefs?
We need to distinguish between
- those that are *harmful*, which we should oppose
- those that are *good* for health, which we should support
- those which are neither harmful nor good for health, which we should tolerate

4 Simple remedies are often the most effective
Drug companies may try to encourage the use of unnecessary, unsafe or unwise medicines. Our aims should be
(i) to choose the most inexpensive and simple but effective remedy for the particular problem (e.g. oral rehydration for diarrhoea instead of expensive antibiotics);
(ii) to encourage people to become independent in their health care by
- using local resources (e.g. personnel, food, medicinal herbs)
- training local people in health care
- educating the local population in self-care
- encouraging local skills and crafts

Professor David Morley suggests that our priorities should be:

- adequate food

- simple health care

- a stimulating environment

The relationship between the environment and certain illnesses

		Malaria	Respiratory infections	Tuberculosis	Gastro-intestinal infections	Helminth infections	Schistosomiasis
Waste disposal	Excreta				⋆	⋆⋆	⋆
	Refuse				⋆		
Water supply	Quality				⋆		⋆
	Quantity				⋆⋆	⋆	⋆⋆
	Bathing/laundry						⋆
Hygiene	Personal hygiene				⋆⋆	⋆	
	Food hygiene				⋆⋆	⋆	
Housing	Standard		⋆	⋆⋆		⋆	
	Over-crowding		⋆⋆	⋆⋆		⋆	
	Poor ventilation		⋆⋆				
	Domestic hygiene			⋆		⋆	
	Atmospheric pollution		⋆⋆				
Vector control	Screening	⋆					
	Surface water drainage	⋆⋆					⋆
	Insecticides Molluscicides Rodenticides	⋆					⋆

⋆ significant relationship
(after Shattock, F. S. 1983)

Typhoid	Measles and infectious diseases	Malnutrition	Scabies and skin diseases	Trachoma	Conjunctivitis	Rodent-borne diseases	Tick-/Flea-borne diseases	Accidents	Infant mortality rate
*		*		*					*
*				*		**			
*		*							*
**		*	**	**	*		*		*
			*						
**				**		*	**		
*		*	**			*			*
		*	*			**	**	**	**
	*	**	**			*	*	**	**
	*		*						
						*	*		
					*				
*				*		**	**		*

* very significant relationship

Abbreviations and symbols used in this series

AC	arm circumference	Hb	haemoglobin
AIDS	acquired immuno-deficiency syndrome	HCG	human chorionic gonadotrophin
		hrly	hourly
AP	antero-posterior	h	hour(s)
APH	antepartum haemorrhage	HVS	high vaginal swab
ARM	artificial rupture of membranes		
		i.e.	that is
BCG	French abbreviation for vaccine for TB	Ig	immunoglobulin
		IM(I)	intramuscular (injection)
BD	twice daily	IU	international units
BP	blood pressure (or, occasionally, biparietal)	IUCD	intra-uterine contraceptive device
		IUD	intra-uterine death
BPD	biparietal diameter	IUGR	intra-uterine growth retardation
BPM/bpm	beats per minute	IV(I)	intravenous (infusion)
BW	birth weight		
		k	kilo (S.I. prefix for 10^3)
°C	degrees centigrade (Celsius)	kg	kilogramme(s)
C	central		
cm	centimetre	l	litre
CNS	central nervous system	Ⓛ	left
CO_2	carbon dioxide	LMP	last menstrual period
cong	congenital	LOA	left occipito-anterior
CPD	cephalo-pelvic disproportion	LOD	left oblique diameter
CSF	cerebro-spinal fluid	LOL	left occipito-lateral
CTG	cardiotocograph	LOP	left occipito-posterior
CXR	chest X-ray	LSA	left sacro-anterior
		L/S/F	length/strength/frequency (of contractions)
dal	decalitre (10 litres)	LSL	left sacro-lateral
dl	decilitre (1/10 litre)	LSP	left sacro-posterior
dpm	drops per minute	LSCS	lower segment Caesarean section
DVT	deep vein thrombosis	LUS	lower uterine segment
D and V	diarrhoea and vomiting		
		m	milli (S.I. prefix for 10^{-3})
E	east	mg	milligramme(s)
ECV	external cephalic version	min	minute(s)
EDD	expected date of delivery	ml	millilitre(s)
e.g.	for example	mm	millimetre(s)
eng	engaged/engagement (of foetal head)	MSU	midstream specimen of urine
		MV	mento-vertical (diameter)
EPA	examination per abdomen (abdominal examination)		
		N	north
EPV	examination per vaginam (vaginal examination)	n	nano (S.I. prefix for 10^{-9})
		NB	note well
ERPC	evacuation of retained products of conception	NG(T)	nasogastric (tube)
ESR	erythrocyte sedimentation rate	O_2	oxygen
etc.	and so on	OD	once daily
EUA	examination under anaesthetic	OF	occipito-frontal (diameter)
		OP	occipito-posterior (diameter)
°F	degrees Fahrenheit	ORS	oral rehydration solution
FH	foetal heart		
		p	pico (S.I. prefix for 10^{-12})
g	gramme	P	pulse (or, occasionally, para)
G	gravida (pregnancy)	PO	orally
GA	general anaesthetic	POP	persistant occipito-posterior
GIT	gastro-intestinal tract	POS/pos	position
GNC	general nursing care	PP	presenting part
G6PD	glucose-6-phosphate dehydrogenase	PPH	post-partum haemorrhage

pres	presentation	U	units
PRN	as necessary	UA	uterine action
PU	pass urine	USSR	Union of Soviet Socialist Republics
PV	per vaginam	UTI	urinary tract infection
QDS	four times daily	UUS	upper uterine segment
®	right	VD	venereal disease
Rx	treatment	Vit	vitamin
RBC	red blood cells		
Resp	respirations	W	west
ROA	right occipito-anterior	WBC	white blood cell
ROD	right oblique diameter	WCC	white blood cell count
ROL	right occipito-lateral	Wk(s)	weeks
ROP	right occipito-posterior		
RSA	right sacro-anterior	>	is greater than
RSL	right sacro-lateral	≥	is greater than or equal to
RSP	right sacro-posterior	<	is less than
		≤	is less than or equal to
S	south	%	per cent
SC	subcutaneous	↓	decreasing/decreased
SCBU	special-care baby unit	↑	increasing/increased
sec	second(s)	→	leads to/leading to
S/E	side effects(s)	+ + +	high degree of (e.g. pain)
SE	south-east	$\overline{52}$	weeks (e.g. $\frac{9}{52}$ = 9 weeks)
SG	specific-gravity	$\overline{12}$	months (e.g. $\frac{9}{12}$ = 9 months)
S.I.	the international system of units	1:5	proportion of 1 in 6
SMB	sub-mento-bregmatic (diameter)	#	fracture
SOB	sub-occipito-bregmatic (diameter)	~	about/approximately
SPA	sub-pubic arch	μ	micro (10^{-6})
stat	immediately	1°	first degree/primary
SWO	stomach wash-out	2°	second degree/secondary
TB	tuberculosis	3°	third degree/tertiary
TDS	three times daily	∴	therefore
T	temperature	♀	female
TLC	tender loving care	♂	male
TOP	termination of pregnancy		

Appendix

Children's dosage of Chloroquine tablets

	1 year	1–3 years	4–6 years	7–12 years	12–15 years
Immediately	½	1	2	2	3–4
At 6 hours	½	¾	1	1	1.5–2
Daily for 3 days	¼	¾	1	1	1.5–2

Normal values

This chart gives ranges of normal values for plasma (P), serum (S), whole blood (B), urine (U) and cerebro-spinal fluid (CSF) levels most commonly used in medical and obstetric practice.

Fluid		S.I. units	Other units	To convert to S.I. units multiply other units by:
P	Bicarbonate	24—32 mmol/l	24—32 mEq/l	No change
P	Bilirubin	5—17 μmol/l	0.3—1.0 mg/100 ml	17.1
B	Blood volume: adult	5 l	—	—
	child	85 ml/kg body weight	—	—
P	Calcium (total)	2.12-2.62 mmol/l	8.5-10.5 mg/100 ml	0.250
B	Carbon dioxide (pCO$_2$)	4.5-6.1 kPa	34-46 mm Hg	0.133
P	Chloride	95-105 mmol/l	95-105 mEq/l	No change
P	Cholesterol	3.6-7.8 mmol/l	140-300 mg/100 ml	0.0259
P	Cortisol	276-690 nmol/l	10-25 μg/100 ml	27.6
P	Creatinine	62-124 μmol/l	0.7-1.4 mg/100 ml	88.4
U	Creatinine	9-17 mmol/24 h	1.0-20 g/24 h	8.84
B	ESR: ♂	3-5 mm/h	—	—
	♀	4-7 mm/h	—	—
	infant	≤ 15 mm/hr	—	—
P	Fibrinogen	1.5-4.0 g/l	150-400 mg/100 ml	0.01
S	Folate	3-20 μg/l	3-20 ng/100 ml	No change
B	Glucose	2.5-4.7 mmol/l	45-85 mg/100 ml	0.0555
B	Haemoglobin:			
	adult	12-14.4 g/dl	12-14.4 g/100 ml	No change
	child	11.5-14.8 g/dl	11.5-14.8 g/100 ml	No change
	newborn	13.6-19.6 g/dl	13.6-19.6 g/100 ml	No change
S	Human placental lactogen (at term)	0.55 μmol/l	10 mg/100 ml	0.055
S	Iron	14-29 μmol/l	80-160 μg/100 ml	0.179
S	Total iron binding capacity	45-72 μmol/l	250-400 μg/100 ml	0.179
B	Lactate	0.14-1.4 mmol/l	3.6-13.0 mg/100 ml	0.111
B	White cell count (Leucocytes)	4.0-11.0 × 10^9/l	4.0-11.0 × 10^3/100 ml	10^6
P	Lipids (total)	4.0-10.0 g/l	400-1000 mg/100 ml	0.01
P	Magnesium	0.7-1.0 mmol/l	1.8-2.4 mg/100 ml	0.411
B	Mean corpuscular haemoglobin (MCH)	27-32 pg	27-32 pg	No change
B	Mean corpuscular haemoglobin concentration (MCHC)	30-35 g/dl	30-35%	No change
B	Mean corpuscular volume (MCV)	75-95 fl	75-95 cu m	No change
U	Oestrogens	60-235 μmol/24 h	—	—
B	Oxygen (pO$_2$)	12-15 kPa	90-110 mmHg	0.133
B	Packed cell volume (PCV)	0.41	41%	0.01
B	pH	7.35-7.45	7.35-7.45	No change
B	Platelets	150-400 × 10^9/l	150,000-400,000/μl	10^6
S	Phenylalanine	42-73 μmol/l	0.7-1.2 mg/100 ml	60.5
P	Phosphate	0.8-1.4 mmol/l	2.5-4.5 mg/100 ml	0.323
P	Potassium	3.8-5.0 mmol/l	3.8-5.0 mEq/l	No change

Fluid		S.I. units	Other units	To convert to S.I. units multiply other units by:
S	Proteins: total	62-80 g/l	6.2-8.2 g/100 ml	10
	albumin	36-52 g/l	3.6-5.2 g/100 ml	10
	globulins	24-37 g/l	2.4-3.7 g/100 ml	10
CSF	Proteins	0.1-0.4 g/l	10-40 mg/100 ml	0.01
B	Red cell count	$4.5 \times 10^{12}/1$	$4.5 \times 10^{6}/\mu 1$	10^6
B	Red cell diameter	6.7-7.7 μm	6.7-7.7 μ	No change
B	Reticulocytes	$10-100 \times 10^9/1$	0.2-2.0%	No change
P	Sodium	136-148 mmol/l	136-148 mEq/l	No change
S	Thyroxine-iodine	244-465 nmol/l	3.1-5.9 μg/100 ml	78.8
B	Urea	2.5-6.6 mmol/l	15-40 mg/100 ml	0.166
P	Vitamin A	0.7-1.7 μmol/l	20-50 μg/100 ml	0.0349
S	Vitamin B_{12}	160-925 ng/μl	160-920 pg/ml	No change

S.I. units

Physical quantity	Name of basic unit	Symbol
length	metre	m
mass	kilogramme	kg
time	second	s
electric current	ampere	A
temperature	kelvin	K
	degrees centigrade (Celsius) is still commonly used	°C
amount of substance	mole	mol
energy	joule	J
force	newton	N
power	watt	W
pressure	pascal	Pa

Prefixes to denote sub-multiples or multiples of the units

Sub-multiple	prefix	symbol
10^{-1}	deci	d
10^{-2}	centi	c
10^{-3}	milli	m
10^{-6}	micro	μ
10^{-9}	nano	n
10^{-12}	pico	p
multiple	prefix	symbol
10^1	deca	da
10^2	hecto	h
10^3	kilo	k
10^6	mega	M

Please note Dosages in this book are usually given 'per kilogramme' (/kg). The dosage can therefore be calculated for any individual whatever the body weight. (This can vary widely depending on the age of the individual and the level of nutrition.) Where dosages are given for an 'adult', it is presumed that the body weight is *50 kg or more*.

Introduction to history-taking and examination

When you have little time and many patients to see, it is tempting not to make the time to take a history of and examine each patient. This may, however, land you in trouble as you may miss something vital.

Even if you cannot do a full examination, be aware of the *whole* person and not just the symptoms with which they present.

And remember ... keep your eyes and ears open *all* the time, even when treatment has started.

General principles

1 Take history first — relatives may be able to give additional information.
2 Examine the patient in as good a light as possible.
3 Examine the patient in a logical order (e.g. starting from the top and working to the bottom of the body) looking at each system in the same order every time you carry out an examination. If you do this you are less likely to miss anything.
4 With children, babies and unconscious patients, your powers of observation need to be even greater.
5 Treat the most life-threatening problem first (e.g. rehydration may be more vital than finding out and treating the cause of the diarrhoea).

     The most vital things to do are:
- maintain an adequate airway
- maintain breathing
- maintain circulation
- stop any bleeding
- maintain hydration

History

Find out the following
- **Symptoms**
  - What are they?
  - Are they present all the time or associated with any particular time or activity?
  - Is there pain? If so, where and what is it like?
- **Onset of illness**
  - Is it chronic?
  - Is it acute?
  - Is it associated with any particular situation, food or other factor?
- **History of any previous illness** in the patient and any treatment given
- **Family history** of any medical problem
- **Diet**
  - What has been eaten today? (especially important if malnutrition is suspected)

Examination

- **General appearance**
  - colour: pale/cyanosed/jaundiced
  - fever
  - state of hydration
  - level of consciousness
  - mental state
  - state of nutrition
- **Cardiovascular system**
  - pulse: rate and regularity
  - blood pressure
  - heart sounds
    (if you are able to use a stethoscope)
  - signs of shock
  - oedema: central or peripheral?
    pitting or non-pitting?
  - raised neck veins
  - signs of anaemia
- **Respiratory system**
  - respirations: rate and type
  - breath sounds
  - intercostal recession or nasal flaring
  - cough: productive? spasms of coughing? etc.
  - sputum: colour and consistency; bloody?
  - chest pain: is it constant; what kind of pain; is it associated with breathing?
  - pleural rub (on auscultation)

- **Head and neck**
  - swellings
  - signs of meningitis
  - signs of injury
  - pain in spine
- **Ear, nose and throat**
  - ears: are they red?
    is there any discharge?
    is patient pulling at ears (sign of pain in ear in child)?
  - throat: signs of infection in the mouth or throat
    any obstruction?
  - nose: bleeding
    obstruction
  - mouth: state of teeth
    tongue — furred/inflamed/dry?
    any ulcers/plaques/spots?
- **Eyes**
  - pain or irritation
  - redness/yellowness
  - disturbed vision
  - failure to close eyes
  - problem with eyelids
  - corneal ulceration/cloudiness
  - pupil size and reaction to light;
    colour of pupil
- **Skin and hair**
  - colour
  - temperature
  - lesions (and lumps)
  - wounds
  - lymphadenopathy
  - infections/infestations
- **Abdomen**
  - size:
    any ascites?
    swelling/lumps?
    is she pregnant?
  - spleen: size
  - tenderness:
    where?
    is it rebound or general tenderness?
  - liver: size

Also find out history of
  - bowel movements: any constipation or diarrhoea?
  - fluid intake and output: any dysuria or haematuria?
                              test urine
  - vomiting
- **Back**
  - pain or tenderness: related to spine;
                        or kidneys?
  - kyphosis or scoliosis
  - swellings
- **Limbs**
  - movement: stiffness/paralysis
  - shape
  - pain
  - muscle wasting
  - varicose veins
- **Chest**
  - pain in ribs
  - intercostal recession
  - unequal movements on left and
    right sides
  - breasts: pain/soreness,
            lumps,
            discharge
- **Genitals**
  - discharge
  - lesions/ulceration/irritation
  - varicose veins of vulva
  - hernia
  - hydrocele

Also look for
- **Loss of sensation** anywhere on the body

For examination of the pregnant woman see THCN Obstetrics

When examining children:
- be gentle and take your time
- allow a parent to hold or be with the child
- ask the parent(s) for history of the illness
- pay special attention to the feeding pattern of the child
- if a procedure is painful, do not say it is not — be honest

Common diseases in the tropics

Malaria

Transmitted by the female anopheline mosquito which
- Breeds in clean, unpolluted water
- Bites at night
- Feeds and rests indoors

} therefore extent of problem depends on:

- Altitude
- Climate
- Housing
- Water sources

Types of malaria	Distribution	Incubation period
Plasmodium falciparum	Africa, Asia, Papua New Guinea and S. America	6–12 days or more
Plasmodium vivax	Especially Asia, S. America (but also Africa)	> 10 days
Plasmodium ovale	Especially Africa	> 10 days
Plasmodium malariae	Worldwide	> 10 days

parasite growing

parasite getting ready to break up

parasite growing

red cell

remains of red cell

parasite going into healthy red cell

parasite breaking up

lots of little parasites ready to go into other red cells

How malaria parasites destroy red cells

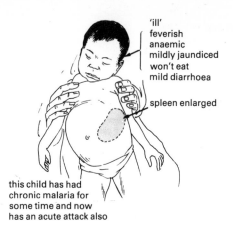

'ill'
feverish
anaemic
mildly jaundiced
won't eat
mild diarrhoea

spleen enlarged

this child has had
chronic malaria for
some time and now
has an acute attack also

A child with malaria

Distinguishing features	Clinical features
• Non-relapsing, • Fever every 48 hours *In stable area:* • Year round transmission • Affects children under 5 • Adults usually immune *In unstable area:* • Seasonal • All ages affected	• Fever and rigours (cold stage → hot stage → sweating) • Headache • D and V • Generalised aches and pains • Pain and enlargement of liver and spleen • Jaundice *Possible complications:* • Anaemia due to haemolysis • Blockage of small blood vessels in brain by sticky RBCs → cerebral malaria (i.e. coma, confusion, delirium, convulsions, death) • Hepatic or renal failure • Pulmonary oedema • Shock • Acute repiratory distress syndrome • Placental insufficiency
• Relapsing • Fever every 3rd day (dormant parasites in liver)	• Cold stage • Hot stage • Sweating
• Relapsing • Fever every 3rd day	• Cold stage • Hot stage • Sweating
• Fever every 4th day (non-relapsing but may occur over 30 years)	As above and • Nephrotic syndrome (children)

Malaria (continued)

Treatment	Prevention	Other possible complications
• 10 mg/kg **Chloroquine** base stat, followed by 5 mg/kg in 6 hours and 5 mg/kg/day for 3 days (1 tablet has 150 mg base) Adult dosage: 4 tablets stat, 2 tablets after 6 hours, 2 tablets daily for 3 days. *If Chloroquine resistance is proven,* give 25 mg/kg/day **Quinine** in 2 divided doses for up to 5 days (depending on the clinical state of the patient) and 26 mg/kg **Fansidar** stat (2 tablets stat). • **For cerebral malaria** — Adults: 5 mg/kg **Chloroquine** base IM 6 hrly for 3 doses; then orally for 2–6 days (but may be given by slow IV infusion over 30 min or more). — Children: 5 mg/kg **Chloroquine** base 6 hrly IM for 3 doses *or* by IVI over 2 hours. If weight not known: give ½ dose × 2 separated by 2 hours. *If Chloroquine resistance is proven,* give 10 mg/kg/day **Quinine** in 2 divided doses by slow IVI, 600 mg 8 hrly PO for 7–14 days. • Use oral route wherever possible, keep IM route for unconscious patients or those who are vomiting • For paediatric oral dosage see Appendix, page 11. *Injections of Chloroquine and Quinine*	*Preventive measures include:* • Giving prophylactic anti-malarials to pregnant women and children under 5 years. — Adults: 25-50 mg/week **Pyrimethamine (Daraprim)** — Children under 10 years: 6.25–18.75 mg/ week **Pyrimethamine** • Residual house spraying to kill mosquitoes using **DDT** (NB DDT needs to be used and stored with great care) • Treatment of breeding sites — search out any clean areas of water, however small (e.g. waterpots, lakes) — for small areas of water cover with a lid or remove water — for larger areas cover with anti-malarial oil	**1 Blackwater fever** This is due to *P. falciparum.* It is associated with irregular use of **Quinine** as a prophylactic. *Clinical features:* • Severe intravascular haemolysis • Haemoglobinuria • Renal failure *Prognosis:* very poor *Differential diagnosis:* In patients with G6PD deficiency and malaria, and taking **Phenacetin**, renal failure is rare. Prognosis is much better as haemolysis usually stops when Hb reaches 6g/dl. **2 Congenital malaria** *Clinical features:* • Irritability • Fever • Lethargy • Anaemia • Jaundice • Hepatosplenomegaly • Diarrhoea • Abdominal distension

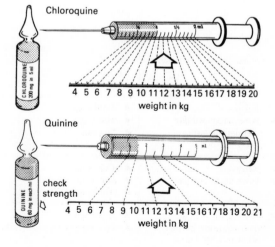

Chloroquine

weight in kg

Quinine

check strength

weight in kg

Anaemia

In developing countries, a 'normal' haemoglobin level may be around 10 g/dl(100 ml).
Therefore, we will classify anaemia (i.e. a haemoglobin level below the accepted norm) as follows:

- Mild to moderate anaemia: 7–10 g/dl
- Moderate to severe anaemia: < 7 g/dl

Causes	Classification and diagnosis	Treatment and prevention
1 **Nutritional deficiency**— iron, folic acid and vitamin C, in particular 2 **Malaria** — anaemia due to RBC haemolysis (see page 17) 3 **Infections** • Hookworm • Trichuriasis (in children) • Schistosomiasis anaemia due to damage to lining of GIT → bleeding (see pages 64–65) • Measles — anaemia due to ulceration of gut → poor absorption 4 **Pregnancy** Anaemia is linked with: • High parity • Continuous state of childbearing • Food taboos • Problems associated with childbearing (see also *THCN Obstetrics*) 5 **Low birth weight** due to prematurity and intra-uterine growth retardation 6 **Abnormal haemoglobins** • Sickle-cell disease (in Afro-Caribbean races) • Thalassaemia (in Mediterranean, Chinese and Indonesian races)	*Diagnosis based on clinical signs and symptoms* • Pallor of mucous membranes, conjunctiva, nailbeds, tongue, palms • Circulatory compensation on exertion • Splenomegaly • Oedema *Laboratory diagnosis* A stock solution of SG 1100 is made by placing 510 g **Crystalline Copper sulphate** in a 4-litre bottle, adding 3018 ml distilled water and shaking repeatedly to ensure complete solution. The stock solution is diluted before use: 47.2 ml made up to 100 ml with water gives an SG of 1048 (standard A) and 41.2 ml made up to 100 ml with water gives an SG of 1042 (standard B). Put 20 ml into each of 5 screw-capped universal containers and use each bottle for no more than 20 tests. A drop of blood taken either from a finger prick or from a venous specimen with a treated pipette is dropped vertically from a height of 1 cm into the solution. After a few seconds the blood will either rise or fall. If the drop of blood rises Hb < 7 g/dl If the drop of blood falls Hb > 10 g/dl If it stays stationary Hb = 7–10 g/dl *Look at the RBCs on a blood slide under the microscope:* If they are small and pale, he/she has iron deficiency If they are larger than normal and pale in the middle, he/she has folic acid or vitamin B_{12} deficiency Otherwise *look for other clinical signs* to indicate cause	• Correct the diet, if necessary, and advise so as to prevent future problems • Treat malaria promptly and give regular antimalarials to children and pregnant women • Kill worms if present (the population may need regular treatment if worms are a common problem) • Give medical treatment: — 20 mg/kg/day **Ferrous sulphate** given in 3 doses until the Hb has been normal for 3 months. Normal adult dosage— 200 mg BD or TDS (for babies, give 12 mg/kg/day syrup in divided doses) — 5–10 mg/day **Folic acid** — blood transfusions only if there is very low cardiac output/ cardiac failure/ pulmonary oedema/ mental confusion Use packed cells and 40 mg **Frusemide** IV (adult) and nurse sitting up

Sickle-cell disease

- Sickle-cell disease is an abnormal form of haemoglobin.
- It is an inherited condition and if both parents are carriers (i.e. if they have sickle-cell trait) then they have a 1 in 4 chance of producing a child with the condition.
- With each pregnancy there is the possibility of one of these outcomes

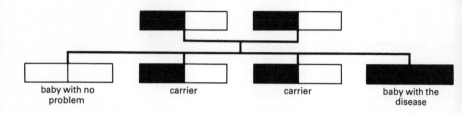

| baby with no problem | carrier | carrier | baby with the disease |

- This condition affects **Afro-Caribbean** races

- The disease causes **chronic anaemia** and **sickling crises** in which the RBC's collapse under stress. **Stress** may be caused by
  - exertion
  - dehydration
  - infection
  - pregnancy
  - general anaesthetic
  - altitude

  but stress of any kind can bring on a sickling crisis.

Common problems

- Becomes obvious 6 months–1 year after birth unless cord blood tests are available for diagnosis
- **Chronic anaemia**
  Fragile cells do not live long
- **Pain**
  Collapsed cells block capillaries. Any major organ or joint can be affected. Often hands and feet are affected first and swell.
- **Enlarged spleen**
  Spleen becomes congested from dealing with damaged RBC's
- **Infection**
  These patients are all very prone to infection
- **Aplastic crisis**
  Bone marrow stops working

Routine care

- Health education to improve general health
- Changes in life-style to prevent a crisis
- Regular check of Hb
- Transfusion of packed cells when in danger
- Supplementation of 5 mg/day **Folic acid**

Maternal/perinatal mortality increased

Increased spontaneous miscarriage/IUGR/foetal distress/stillbirth and difficult delivery from pelvic deformities leading to birth injury

Management of sickling crisis

- Admit to hospital
- Search for cause
- Give broad-spectrum **Antibiotic**
- Give adequate pain relief
- Check hydration and push fluid intake
- Transfusion of packed cells

Thalassaemia

- This is another form of abnormal haemoglobin
- It is an inherited condition like sickle-cell disease. As in sickle-cell disease if both parents are carriers there is a 1:3 chance of producing a baby with the disease (see previous page)
- Alpha thalassaemia affects Indonesian, Chinese and Greek races
- Beta thalassaemia affects people from Mediterranean countries

Alpha thalassaemia

- Alpha thalassaemia major
  A child born with this disease will die perinatally as there is no foetal Hb
- Profound anaemia leads to intra-uterine death/still birth/or perinatal death

Beta thalassaemia

- Beta thalassaemia major
  A child born with this disease does produce some foetal Hb
- The child will present at 3-6 months with
  — profound anaemia
  — enlarged liver and spleen
- The child will die unless regular blood transfusion can be given 4-6 weekly, throughout life
- Multiple blood transfusions can lead to iron overload so give: 2-4 g **Desferrioxamine** SC over 12 hours, 6 nights a week from the second year of life, with 200 mg/day **Ascorbic acid**, to increase iron excretion

Cardiac and respiratory diseases

Examination of the patient

This should include the following:

- *History of the illness*
- *Pulse*
  - rate:
    normal adult, 60–80 per min (↑ in pregnancy)
    normal child, 80–100 per min
    normal baby, 100–140 per min
  - regularity
- *Blood pressure*
  - normal
  - high (diastolic > 90 mm Hg)
  - low (systolic < 90 mm Hg)
- *Neck veins*
  - normal
  - raised (as in heart failure)

Disease	General notes	Pathology and aetiology	Diagnosis
Congestive cardiac failure	Most common causes are • Severe anaemia • Hypertension	• The output of the heart is inadequate for the needs of the tissues and organs → fluid retention in either the lungs (most commonly) or the systemic veins and liver causing peripheral oedema	• Clinical picture

- *Respiration*
  - rate:
    normal adult, 12-20 per min
    normal child, < 30 per min
    normal baby, < 40 per min
  - type of breathing:
    normal, easy and regular; or shallow; or deep; or laboured/difficult (dyspnoea)/painful?
  - does the breath smell?
  - is there a wheeze on expiration?
  - is there inspiratory stridor (i.e. noisy breathing)?
  - is there flaring of the nostrils on inspiration? (normally nostrils do not move)
  - is there intercostal recession (i.e. is the skin sucked in between the ribs and at the angle of the neck on inspiration?) If so, there is obstruction of some kind or infection.
  - is there a cough? If so, is it dry (like a dog's bark) or wet (with sputum coughed up)? Is sputum yellow, green, bloodstained or frothy?
  - is there a whoop?
  - does the chest wall move equally on both sides on inspiration?

Also look for the following symptoms

- *Cyanosis*

(especially around the lips and conjunctiva—a serious sign)

- *Oedema*

Press thumb firmly and slowly over lower end of the tibia for 5 sec. If a mark is left, oedema is present. Also look at the face, sacrum and fingers.

Clinical features	Treatment	Prevention
<ul><li>Body weakness</li><li>Cough</li><li>Chest pains on exertion</li><li>Oedema of legs and/or abdomen (visible as 'pitting')</li><li>Raised neck veins</li><li>Fast pulse — triple rhythm</li><li>Mild proteinuria</li><li>Ascites is possible</li><li>Rapid weight gain in infants (due to fluid retention)</li><li>Dyspnoea on exertion</li></ul>	<ul><li>Patients should rest, sitting up; make sure that complications of bedrest do not occur</li><li>If cardiac arrhythmia is present give 0.5-0.7 mg **Digoxin** by slow IV injection and repeat after 4-6 hours; maintain with 0.25-0.5 mg daily (0.03-0.06 mg/kg/day for children)</li><li>Give a diuretic: 40-80 mg/day **Frusemide** PO (1-4 mg/kg/day for children) and change to 5-10 mg **Bendrofluazide** daily as condition improves If oedema is severe, give 40 mg **Frusemide** by *slow* IV injection (1-2 mg/kg/day)</li><li>Encourage eating of citrus fruits to provide **Potassium**</li><li>Correct any cause of heart failure such as anaemia and hypertension</li></ul>	<ul><li>Take regular exercise</li><li>Eat a less refined diet</li><li>Treat anaemia</li></ul>

Cardiac and respiratory diseases (continued)

Disease	General notes	Pathology and aetiology	Diagnosis
Hypertension	• May be 2° to renal or endocrine disorders, or the cause may be unknown	• ↑ peripheral resistance • If untreated → arteriosclerosis and cardiac failure	• ↑ BP, diastolic > 90 mm Hg • Clinical picture
Rheumatic fever	• Associated with poor socio-economic conditions	• Caused by β haemolytic streptococcus	• Clinical picture • History of sore throat
Pneumonia	• Very common • Usually bacterial • May be 2° to measles	• Bacterial *or* viral	• Clinical picture • CXR
Bronchitis	• Common	• Bacterial	• Clinical picture

Clinical features	Treatment	Prevention
• ↑ BP • Headache ⎫ • Dizziness ⎬ if severe • Loss of energy and fatigue • Eye changes (use an ophthalmoscope)	• Patients should rest • Give 5–10 mg/kg/day **Bendrofluazide** PO *or* 40 mg **Propranolol** PO BD (more expensive) *or* 10 mg TDS **Debrisoquine** (more expensive)	• As for congestive cardiac failure
• Tachycardia • Mitral systolic murmur • Jugular venous pressure ↑ • Hepatomegaly • Pain in joints; pain moves from one joint to another and is associated with swelling, redness and heat • Curved red lines or lumps under the skin • History of sore throat	• Give 20 mg/kg/day **Penicillin** in divided doses • **Aspirin** taken with milk or Sodium bicarbonate • Watch carefully for signs of heart damage	• Treat streptococcal sore throat promptly with **Penicillin**
• Cough (painful) • ↑ respiratory rate • Indrawing (intercostal recession) • Flaring of nostrils • Fever • Cyanosis	• Give 150–300 mg **Benzyl Penicillin** IM 6 hrly (divided doses) for one day then 300 mg **Procaine Penicillin** IM daily (divided doses) • Give **Oxygen** PRN, if available *If the patient is not improving after 2–3 days:* • Take CXR and look for — signs of TB — staphlococcal infection (cysts in lungs: Rx **Cloxacillin**) *If 2° to measles:* • Give 50–100 mg/kg/day **Chloramphenicol** *or* 30 mg/kg/day **Benzyl Penicillin**	
• Productive cough • ↑ respiratory rate (40–60 breaths/min) • Fever • Yellow or green sputum • Wheeze	• Treat fever by removing clothing and by tepid sponging (if necessary) • If fever > 38.0°C, give **Aspirin** • If high fever (> 38.5°C), give **Penicillin** or **Sulphadimidine**	

Cardiac and respiratory diseases (continued)

Disease	General notes	Pathology and aetiology	Diagnosis
'Croup' (Laryngitis)	• Usually bacterial but may be due to diphtheria, so look for the membrane of diphtheria in the throat (see page 82)	• Mucosa of airway swells → obstruction	• Clinical picture
Asthma	• Recurrent attacks • Generally worse in children and improves as they get older • Caused by allergy • Generally worse at certain times of the year • May be associated with eczema • Anxiety may increase the problem	• Allergy → swelling of mucous membranes in respiratory tract → difficulty in breathing	• Clinical picture • History of repeated attacks
Whooping cough	(see page 82)		
TB	(see page 28)		
Anaemia	(see page 19)		
Diabetic coma	(see page 32)		
Anaphylactic shock	• Caused by an allergy to food, medicine, vaccination etc. (especially anti-snake venom serum or tetanus antitoxin)		

Clinical features	Treatment	Prevention
• Dry cough • Stridor on inspiration • Indrawing (intercostal recession) • Flaring of nostrils • Laboured breathing	• Give **Chloramphenicol** for the infection • Fill the room with steam or hang wet cloths near to the patient so that the air is moist (i.e. humidify the air) • Perform tracheostomy if cyanosis continues (*ideally this should be done by a doctor*)	
• Wheeze on expiration • Intercostal recession • Flaring of nostrils	• Humidify the air • If mild, give 1 mg/kg **Ephedrine** TDS *or* 3 mg/kg **Theophylline** PO 6 hrly • If severe, give 0.5 ml **Adrenaline** SC or IM (0.3 ml for children 7–12 years, 0.25 ml for children 1–6 years) Do not give to babies under 1 year If necessary, repeat the dose after 30 min and 2 hours. *Never* give more than 3 doses. *OR* 250 mg **Aminophylline** IV over 5–10 min 8 hrly (adult dose) • Watch pulse—if ↑ 30 bpm or more, do not give any more drugs	
• Dyspnoea • ↓ consciousness • Dehydration • Deep, rapid breathing		
• Dyspnoea—acute onset • Wheeze • Cold, sweating skin • Fast, weak pulse • Low blood pressure • Acute onset of skin rash or swellings • Fever • Oedema of face or eyes • ↓ consciousness	• Give **Adrenaline** SC or IM (Dosage as for asthma) • Give 25–50 mg **Promethazine** IM (12.5–25 mg for children 7–12 years, 6–12 mg for children 1–6 years, 2.5 mg for babies under 1 year) Repeat after 2–4 h if necessary *or* 30–50 mg **Diphenhydramine** (10–30 mg for children, 5 mg for babies) Repeat after 2–4 h if necessary	• Watch patient for 30 min after giving injection of anti-snake venom etc. for signs of shock

Tuberculosis

- Caused by *Mycobacterium tuberculosis* via
  - droplet infection from another infected person
  - milk
  - skin and mucous membranes of another infected person
- Associated with
  - poverty
  - undernutrition
  - concurrent disease (e.g. measles)
  - overcrowding
- Peak age in developing countries is under 5 years

Primary Lesion

Commonly in lung periphery:
- Area of inflammatory exudate
- Caseation and cavitation
- May ulcerate into pleural sac →
  empyema
- May spread to lymph nodes draining area

Clinical features possible:
(occur 4–8 weeks after infection)
- Febrile illness
- Erythema nodosum
- 'Red eye'—phlyctenular conjunctivitis
- Supraclavicular lymphadenopathy

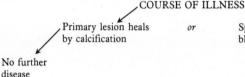

COURSE OF ILLNESS

Primary lesion heals *or* Spread via
by calcification bloodstream

No further Secondary TB lesions
disease (see below)

Secondary Lesions

- **Adult TB Lung** (≥ $\frac{3}{52}$ after 1° infection)

  Clinical features:
  - cough for > $\frac{4}{52}$
  - haemoptysis
  - fever and night sweats
  - weight loss and anorexia
  - supraclavicular lymphadenopathy

  Diagnosis:
  - sputum for microscopy: acid fast
    bacilli seen
  - gastric aspiration (child)
  - HEAF test, but may be negative
    falsely in measles; kwashiorkor;
    miliary TB; or TB meningitis etc.
  - CXR: collapse/pneumonia/pleural
    effusion

- **TB Renal Tract** (peak age: 20–45 years)

  Clinical features:
  - frequency, dysuria and haematuria
  - loin pain and renal colic

  Diagnosis:
  - urine for microscopy

- **Miliary TB** (Insidious onset—prone
  to occur after measles)

  Clinical features:
  - unwell, febrile child
  - weight loss
  - dyspnoea and cyanosis
  - hepatosplenomegaly
  - lymphadenopathy

  Diagnosis:
  - CXR: hazy, white dots over lung
    fields
  - Eye: tubercular dots seen with
    opthalmoscope

- **TB Abdomen**

  Clinical features:
  - ascites
  - wasting
  - pain
  - salpingitis → infertility ⎤ may be
                                ⎬ sexually
  - epididymitis in men   ⎦ transmitted

- *TB Meningitis* ($\leq \frac{6}{12}$ of 1° infection)

  Clinical features:
  — anorexia
  — lethargy
  — irritability and mood changes
  — vomiting
  — headache (becomes constant)
  — constipation
  — abdominal pain
  — tense fontanelle (in child)

  May deteriorate to:
  — convulsions
  — opisthotonus
  — papilloedema
  — coma
  — death

  Diagnosis:
  Lumbar puncture for CSF
  — ↑ protein
  — ↓ glucose
  — lymphocytes + +
  — forms cobweb clot when allowed to stand

- *TB Skin* (develops slowly, recurrent)
  — painless chronic patches, sores, ulcers or big warts
  — painless disfiguring tumours

- *TB Bone (spine and long bones)*

  Clinical features:
  — local pain and tenderness (especially in 10th and 11th thoracic vertebrae); pain relieved by rest
  — angulation
  — paraplegia due to destruction of bone

  Diagnosis:
  — AP and lateral X-ray of spine (or relevant bones)

- *TB Lymph Glands*
  — rubbery glands (especially in neck)
  — soften
  — may form sinus
  — recurrent
  — painless

Treatment

Principles of treatment

1 Always use at least 2 drugs
2 If TB lung use at least 3 drugs for 2-3 months, then 2 drugs for the rest of the time
3 Treat for $\frac{12}{12}$; if TB meningitis, treat for 2 years
4 In TB meningitis, give 10 mg **Hydrocortisone** daily intrathecally for 5 days, then 2 mg/kg/day **Prednisolone** PO for $\frac{2}{52}$ and 10 mg/day **Pyridoxine**

Dosages of drugs

Isoniazid (INAH)   10-20 mg/kg/day PO (this should be based on weight of the child); also give **Pyridoxine**
Thiacetazone   5-10 mg/kg/day PO (very cheap but problems with resistance)
Streptomycin   20-40 mg/kg/day IM for $\frac{3}{52}$-$\frac{4}{52}$ (S/E deafness) (adult — 1 g IM daily)
P.A.S.   250 mg/kg/day PO (S/E rash) (10-12 g daily — adult)
Ethambutol   15-25 mg/kg/day PO (do not use for renal TB) (S/E optic atrophy)
Rifampicin   8-12 mg/kg/day PO (expensive) (S/E jaundice and hepatosplenomegaly) (450-600 mg daily — adult)
Pyrazinamide   20-30 mg/kg/day PO

Suggested regimes

1 **Isoniazid**
  Thiacetazone
  Streptomycin
  Pyridoxine
  } Daily for $\frac{2}{12}$, then **Thiazina** for $\frac{12}{12}$

2 **High dose Isoniazid**
  Streptomycin
  Pyridoxine
  } Daily for $\frac{2}{12}$, then twice a week for 1 year

3 **Isoniazid**
  Pyrazinamide
  Ethambutol
  or **Streptomycin**
  Rifampicin
  Pyridoxine
  } Daily for $\frac{6}{12}$ ★

★(Expensive therefore only use if resistance proven to other drugs)

Prevention

- Give 0.1 ml **BCG** intradermally; stimulates cell mediated response therefore child's nutritonal status must be good; varying results obtained from studies of effectiveness
- Treat a pregnant woman who has TB immediately (avoid **Streptomycin**); she can breast-feed her baby after 3-4 weeks of treatment

  Give baby — BCG
  — **Isoniazid** for $\frac{6}{12}$ - $\frac{12}{12}$
- Improve diet, housing, etc.

Disturbed consciousness, fits and epilepsy

Examination of the patient

This should include all of the following:

- *History of illness*
  - from patient or relatives
- *General observation of*
  - temperature
  - pulse
  - blood pressure
  - respiration
  } (see pages 14–15)
- *Signs of dehydration*
  - reduced skin elasticity
  - dry mouth
  - sunken eyes
  - signs of shock
  - sunken fontanelle in infants
  } (see pages 54–55)
- *Signs of shock*
  - low blood pressure: systolic < 90 mm Hg
  - rapid pulse
  - pale, sweating skin
- *Neck stiffness*
  - bend head towards chest: there should not normally be any pain or stiffness

Condition	Diagnosis	Clinical features
Meningitis Adults and older children	• Clinical picture • Lumbar puncture and examine CSF — does it turn cloudy when Pandy's solution added? — examine for cells, protein and bacteria	• Headache • Mental confusion • Vomiting • Drowsiness • Fever • Photophobia • Neck stiffness • ↓ consciousness } acute onset within hours unless TB meningitis
Infants	• Clinical picture • Lumbar puncture	• Poor feeding • Vomiting • Fits • Non-pulsatile, bulging fontanelle • Skin rash or bruising • Twitching of limbs Young babies rarely have neck stiffness

- *Fontanelle in infants*
  - should *not* bulge unless child cries
  - should pulsate
- *Mental state*
  - is patient confused?
- *Kernig's sign (in children, not in adults or small babies):*
  - you should be able to straighten child's leg without causing pain. If it causes pain, it is abnormal.
- *Pupil reaction*
  - are the pupils equal in size?
  - do they react to light?
    i.e. ↓ size with ↑ light
    　　↑ size with ↓ light
- *Level of consciousness*
  - fully conscious and alert
  - drowsy: responds to orders
  - responds to pain (e.g. if pricked with a pin) but not to orders, otherwise unconscious
  - responds only to very severe pain (press heel tendon hard between thumb and forefinger): patient will move leg or show pain on face, but otherwise unconscious
  - unconscious: makes no response, even to severe pain

These observations need to be repeated regularly and recorded with date and time.

Treatment	Prevention
<ul><li>500 mg **Ampicillin** (adult) IM 6 hrly (100-300 mg/kg/day) *or* 1 000 000 units **Crystalline Penicillin** IM 6 hrly</li><li>Also 50-100 mg/kg/day **Chloramphenicol** in 3 divided doses for young children and if causative organism unknown</li><li>Lower fever by — tepid sponging — **Aspirin**</li><li>If any possibility of TB meningitis, give 20 mg/kg/day **Streptomycin** IM (see pages 28-29)</li><li>Exclude other infection (e.g. measles, mumps, etc.) and treat as necessary</li><li>Maintain airway and circulation ⎫</li><li>IVI, for nutrition, and/or NG tube feeds ⎪</li><li>Nurse semi-prone　　　　　　　　　 *NB*</li><li>Suction, as necessary　　　　 ⎬ *as for any*</li><li>Catheter — closed drainage　　 *unconscious*</li><li>Turn 2 hrly to avoid pressure sores *patient*</li><li>Observations as at top of pages ⎭</li></ul>	<ul><li>BCG vaccination</li><li>Measles vaccination</li></ul>

Disturbed consciousness, fits and epilepsy (continued)

Condition	Diagnosis	Clinical features
Diabetic coma	• Clinical picture • Blood glucose levels, found by testing with Dextrostix, show high levels • Glucose and ketones are found in the urine	• Weight loss • Thirst • Passing urine + + + • Abdominal pain • Drowsiness and ↓ consciousness • Dehydration • Rapid, deep breathing • Sugar and ketones in the urine • Breath smells of acetone • May be signs of other infection • Rapid, weak pulse
Hypoglycaemia	• Clinical picture • Low blood glucose levels	• Body weakness and faintness • Mental confusion • Fits • Acts like someone who is 'drunk' • Responds to being given glucose • May be a known diabetic In a baby: • Poor feeding • Twitching
Cerebral malaria	• Clinical picture • Blood film shows malarial parasites + + +	• Fever • Fits • Headache • Mental confusion or abnormal behaviour • Neck stiffness • Urine normal Especially common cause of coma in children
Head injury	• History of injury • Clinical picture	• ↓ consciousness • Fits • Vomiting • Incontinence • Mental confusion or abnormal behaviour
Brain haemorrhage	• Clinical picture	• Sudden onset of ↓ consciousness or fits • Sudden onset of weakness or paralysis of limbs, difficulty in talking, incontinence • ↑ BP • Fever (?) • Urine normal
Dehydration	• Clinical features	• Signs of dehydration (see page 55) • ↓ consciousness

Treatment	Prevention
• Give 10 units soluble **Insulin** immediately IM. Repeat with 5 units IM hrly until blood glucose is 10–16 mmol/l. Monitor blood glucose level carefully and repeat **Insulin** (SC) and adjust dosage as necessary. • IVI to replace fluid deficit. Start with 0.9% Normal **saline** or, if acidotic, isotonic **Sodium bicarbonate** (Sodium hydrogen carbonate) or **Hartmann's solution.** May need to give 3 litres. Then give up to 2 litres 5% **Dextrose.** Then continue 5% **Dextrose** and give necessary **Insulin.** • Use **Potassium** supplements • Care for the unconscious patient	• Keep to prescribed diet and avoid sugar, sweets and refined foods • Reassess **Insulin** needs
• Give 50 ml 50% **Glucose** IV, repeat as necessary • Monitor the blood glucose levels carefully • If the patient is a diabetic, be ready to reassess **Insulin** needs, adjust diet, advise on timing of meals etc. after he/she recovers • Care for the unconscious patient	• If diabetic, carefully monitor **Insulin** intake and keep to diet • In babies, feed as soon as possible after birth. Give special attention to babies of diabetic mothers
• Give adults 5 mg/kg **Chloroquine** base 6 hrly IM for 3 doses. Then orally for 2–6 days *or* IVI over 30 min or more • Give children dosage as for adult but if it is put in IVI give over 2 hours • If Chloroquine resistance: give 10 mg/kg/day **Quinine** in 2 divided doses by slow IVI	• Malaria prophylaxis for children and pregnant women (see page 18)
• Observe closely until regain consciousness • X-ray to exclude # skull or spine and treat accordingly • Care for the unconscious patient	
• Observe closely • Maintain airway by positioning patient in recovery position (on side with head down) • Prevent pressure sores and contractures of limbs by 2 hrly turning and passive movements	• Treat patients with hypertension
• Correct dehydration by use of IV fluids or oral fluids or NG fluids • Diagnosis of cause and treat accordingly (e.g. infection, cholera)	

Disturbed consciousness, fits and epilepsy (continued)

Condition	Diagnosis	Clinical features
Alcohol intoxication	• Clinical features	• ↓ consciousness • Confusion or abnormal behaviour
Eclampsia	• Clinical features • History of pregnancy	• Oedema • Proteinuria • Epigastric pain • Headache • Visual disturbances • Fits • Coma • ↑ BP
Tetanus	• Clinical features • History of injury?	• Muscular spasm • Fits
Febrile convulsion	• Childhood, typically $\frac{6}{12}$-4 years • High fever or sudden rise in fever	• Fit • Fever • Signs of other infection
Epilepsy 'Grand mal'	• Clinical features • History of repeated fits *Causes:* • No known cause • Head injury • Meningitis • Cerebral tumour or abcess	• ↓ consciousness • Incontinence • Tongue bitten • Fits usually followed by sleep; fits not induced by noise or movement

Some other causes of fits and/or disturbed consciousness

- African trypanosomiasis
- American trypanosomiasis
- Relapsing fever
- Scrub typhus
} (see pages 72-77)
- Liver failure which is 2° to cirrhosis or hepatitis or cancer
- Renal failure which is 2° to schistosomiasis or streptococcal glomerulonephritis
- Hydatid cyst in brain
- Poisoning
- Hypo-or hypernatraemia — especially in babies

Treatment	Prevention
• Encourage the patient to drink fluids when conscious • Await recovery • Exclude other causes meanwhile	• Avoid alcohol abuse
(See *THCN Obstetrics*)	(See *THCN Obstetrics*)
See pages 84–85	• Vaccination
• Lower fever by tepid sponging, removing clothes, giving **Aspirin** or **Paracetamol** • Give **Antibiotics** or **Antimalarials** depending on cause of fever • Give 3-6 mg/kg/day **Phenobarbitone** IM in 3 divided doses or PO for 3 days to stop fits	• Malaria prophylaxis • Vaccination to prevent infectious diseases • Health education for mother as to how to lower fever in child
• *If fits still occurring:* Give 3-10 mg/kg **Phenobarbitone** injection IM once. If still fitting after 15 min, repeat dose *once* *or* 0.1-0.2 mg/kg **Paraldehyde** IM and repeat *once* after 15 min if still fitting If fits still continue: give 5-10 mg **Diazepam** (Valium) by *slow* IV injection (adults) • To prevent further fits: give 3-6 mg/kg/day **Phenobarbitone** in 3 divided doses • Care for the unconscious patient • Protect from injury during fit by moving onto floor away from furniture, fire etc. • Ensure that there is no physical cause for the fits that can be treated	

Eye diseases

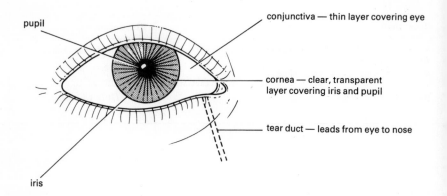

Normal healthy eye

- Examine all patients in a good light
- Blindness and poor vision is common in the developing world and much of this could be prevented

Condition	General notes	Clinical features
Conjunctivitis	May be due to: - Bacterial infection - Viral infection (e.g. measles) - Allergy (as in hay fever)	- Irritation and discharge, usually in both eyes - Swollen eyelids - Vision normal
Foreign body	- History of something getting into the eye	- Pain and irritation in one eye - Conjunctivitis - Vision normal - Foreign body seen in the eye
Phlyctenular conjunctivitis	- Mostly found in children - Symptom of TB	- Small (1–2 mm), yellow swelling on sclera near the cornea - Painful - Conjunctiva red near it - Eyes watering + +
Gonococcal ophthalmitis (Ophthalmia neonatorum)	- Found in children of mothers who have untreated gonorrhoea - Emergency as it may cause sight loss	- Red, swollen eyes in 1st 2 days of life - Discharge + +

Examination of the eye:

- *History of onset of problem and/or trauma to eye*
- *Change in visual ability*
  - ↓ vision
  - blurring
  - spots before eyes
- *Movement of eyes*
  - normal
  - jerky
  - squint
- *Discharge from eye*
  - watering + +
  - pus
- *Pain or irritation in eye(s)*
- *Colour of conjunctiva*
  - normal
  - red
  - yellow

If **ophthalmoscope** used: can also look at retina and inner parts of eye

- *Iris*
  - signs of inflammation
- *Pupils*
  - of equal size?
  - reaction to light
  - clear or opaque
- *Cornea*
  - transparent or dull
  - white/grey spot or line
  - scarring
  - line of pus behind
- *Eyelids*
  - able to close
  - swelling
  - eyelashes growing in
  - follicles under upper eyelid
- *Eyebrows*
  - present or absent

	Treatment	Prevention
swollen eyelid / conjunctiva red	• Clean eyes 4 hrly • Apply **Chlortetracycline** eye ointment QDS • If eyelids swollen, give **Penicillin** PO • If measles, give **Vit A** • If allergy, no treatment needed	• Keep eyes clean • Give measles vaccination
	• Remove foreign body with corner of a clean cloth, *or* wash out with **saline** eye bath	
small yellow swelling / red conjunctiva near swelling	• Treat TB and this will then clear • Reassure the mother • Pain relief, as necessary	• Give BCG vaccination
	• Give 150 000 units **Crystalline Penicillin** BD for 3 days IM • Give **Penicillin** eye drops every 10 min for 1 hour; then every hour for 6 hours; then every 2-3 hours for 3 days • Clean eyes regularly	• In endemic area: put 1 drop of 1% **Silver nitrate** solution once only into each eye at birth of all babies • Treat mothers antenatally • Wipe baby's eyes immediately at delivery

Eye diseases (continued)

Condition	General notes	Clinical features
Trachoma	• Chronic conjuctivitis which takes years to develop • If treated before corneal damage, normal vision can be retained • Spread by touch or flies	• Red, watery eyes • Small red or grey follicles on inside of the upper eyelid • Grey appearance or white scarring of the cornea • Scarring of the eyelids • Eyelashes turn in and irritate the eye • ↓ vision
Xerophthalmia (Vitamin A deficiency)	• Often associated with measles and/or malnutrition • Will cause blindness if untreated	See pages 90–93 • Cornea dull and dry • Bitot's spots • Cornea opaque, soft and ulcerated, if untreated i.e. keratomalacia
Corneal ulcer	• May be due to — trauma — Vit A deficiency — infection (e.g. trachoma) — onchocerciasis — leprosy: due to exposure as person unable to close his/her eyes	• History of trauma to eye • Pain or irritation in one eye • Photophobia • Dull cornea with white/grey spot on it • ↓ vision Infection may spread behind the eye → **hypopyon** i.e. pus behind cornea, this needs urgent treatment
Iritis	• May be caused by local or general infection or toxoplasmosis • May be auto-immune reaction	• Blurred vision • Pain + + • Redness around cornea (iris) • Pupil small and irregular • Eyes watering + + • Photophobia
Cataract	• May be congenital (as in congenital rubella syndrome) • More often, associated with old age • Lens of eye becomes cloudy	• Pupil looks grey or white when light shines on it • ↓ vision
Glaucoma	• Due to ↑ intraocular pressure • May be acute or chronic onset	• Pupil in the affected eye is bigger and has no reaction to light • ↓ vision, especially laterally • Redness round cornea and iris • Eyeball in affected eye feels harder than the other one • Headache } if acute onset • Vomiting }

	Treatment	Prevention
follicles under lid, grey cloudy cornea or white scarring, white of eye slightly inflamed	• Apply **Chlortetracycline** eye ointment BD for 5 days each month, for 6 months • Keep eyes clean	• Wash eyes regularly
Bitot's spot, cornea dull, conjunctiva folded	• Apply **Chloretracycline** ointment • Give **Vit A** injections • Keep clean (see pages 90–93)	• Good balanced diet with foods rich in **Vit A**
inflammation worst next to cornea, white or grey spot or line on cornea	• Apply **Chlortetracycline** eye ointment TDS • Keep eyes clean • Give **Vit A**, if endemic Vit A deficiency area • If due to exposure due to leprosy, stitch eyelids together	• Prevent **Vit A** deficiency • Keep eyes clean • Treat infection promptly • Surgery on eyes of leprosy patients to enable them to shut eyelids
pupil small and may be irregular, inflammation around cornea	• Use topical **Steroid** drops or ointment • Use **Atropine** (to relieve pain and discourage adhesions) • Warmth • Cover eye	
	• Surgery • Strong glasses, after surgery	• Immunise against rubella before pregnancy
pupil bigger, inflammation. *Normal eye* *Affected eye*	• Use **Pilocarpine** eye drops 4 hrly • Give diuretic **Acetazolamide (Diamox)** • Best treated by surgery	

Eye diseases (continued)

Condition	General notes	Clinical features
Onchocerciasis 'River blindness'	• Caused by *Onchocerca volvulus* transmitted by *Simulium* blackfly (see page 62) • Causes blindness	• Redness • Eye watering + + • Iritis • Dull, pitted cornea—sclerosing keratitis • Corneal scarring • Inflamed retina/choroid • Optic nerve damage
Stye	• Infection of gland surrounding eyelash	• Red lump on eyelid • Swollen eyelid
Pterygium		• Fleshy growth which grows out from edge of eye towards the cornea • Aggravated by wind, dust and sunlight
Squint (Strabismus)	• If the squinting eye is not used, it gets weaker and cannot be used	
Leprosy	• Exposure 2° to eyelid muscles weakness • Damage to eye 2° to corneal insensitivity • Inflammation of eye which leads to adhesions • Glaucoma 2° to inflammation • Infiltration of eye by *Mycobacterium*	• See corneal ulcer • See corneal ulcer • Pain • Photophobia • Blurred vision • Watery eye • Eyeball tenderness • See glaucoma • Small white opacities on iris

Some other conditions affecting eyes

- Thyrotoxicosis
- Burns or liquids coming in contact with the eye
- Tribal medicines
- *Herpes simplex* and *Herpes zoster*
- Cerebro-vascular accident/brain haemorrhage
- Eclampsia (see *THCN Obstetrics*) causes disturbance of vision
- Detached retina which is 2° to injury to eye — causes sudden onset of spots in front of the eyes
- Diabetes
- Hypertension

	Treatment	Prevention
	• Must give 100 mg **Suramin** to kill adult worms • **DEC** (see pages 62–63) to kill microfilariae • ?**Corticosteroid** eye drops	• Treat promptly and effectively • See pages 62–63 for further measures
stye	• Apply **Chlortetracycline** eye ointment TDS • If eyelid very swollen give **Penicillin** injections	• Keep eyes clean
pterygium	• Surgery to remove it before it reaches the pupil • Protect the eyes with sunglasses	
	• Keep the good eye covered with a patch until the other eye stays straight.	
	• See corneal ulcer • See corneal ulcer • Warm compresses to eye • Analgesics • Keep affected eyes shaded • Refer to opthalmologist • Treat leprosy	

Skin conditions

Some definitions of skin lesions

Macule	flat lesion
Papule	raised lesion
Vesicle	lesion filled with a clear liquid
Pustule	lesion filled with pus
Cellulitis	inflammation of tissues around a lesion

1   Caused by bacterial infection

Condition	Site	Description of lesion
Impetigo	• Face • Nose • Ears • Head • Buttocks	• Progress from macule to papule to vesicle to pustule, then they break and yellow crusts form • Can cause septicaemia or osteomyelitis in severe cases • Especially serious in a young baby
Boils and abcesses	• Anywhere	• Papular • Pustular
Pyoderma	• Anywhere, it may be 2° infection of bite, scabies, cut etc.	• Pustular • May be inflamed
Ulcers	• 90% are below the knee	• Irregular shape • Red, swollen and tender • Slightly raised edge • Floor of ulcer covered in pus
Syphilis	• Genitals • (Mouth or anus)	• Painless blister or open sore • Lasts a few days and then disappears, but disease continues • Followed by rash over body or itchy rash over hands or feet, fever, sore throat, mouth sores, swollen joints—it may be weeks or months later that these symptoms occur • If untreated heart disease, paralysis, insanity etc.
Lymphogranuloma	• Groin • Anus • Genitals	• Lumps and lymph nodes in groin open up and drain pus, heal, then open again • Painful, oozing sores in anus

Some questions to ask when taking a history

- Where are the lesions?
- How big are the lesions?
- What shape are they?
- What colour are they?
- Are they flat or raised?
- Are they symmetrically situated on the body?

- Are they solid or filled with liquid?
- Do they have a well-defined edge?
- Are they itchy?
- Are they wet or dry?
- Are there any other symptoms?

Treatment	Prevention
• Wash the lesions with soap and water • Bath in **Hypochlorite** or **Permanganate** solution • Dry, then apply **Gentian Violet** or **Chlortetracycline** ointment to lesions • Give **Penicillin** (longacting) if infection speading or child under 1 year	
• Hot compresses (do not burn patient) • Give **Penicillin** if cellulitis, or fever, or many boils • If necessary, lance boil when lesion feels fluid and the top is thin. Leave open to drain, packing it with wet dressing	
• Soak with **Hypochlorite** or **Permanganate** solution • Apply **Gentian Violet** or **Chlortetracycline** ointment to lesion after drying	• Keep any broken skin clean
• Remove pus and clean with **Hydrogen peroxide** or **Hypochlorite** solution • If small, apply dry dressing • If large, apply dressing soaked in **Hypochlorite** solution and renew daily • Give **Procaine Penicillin** IM daily for 3-7 days	
• Give 600 000-1 million units per day **Procaine Penicillin** for 12 days *or* • Give 750 mg **Tetracycline** QDS for 10 days • Treat all sexual contacts	• Avoid indiscriminate sex • Get prompt treatment • Treat all contacts
• Give 250-500 mg **Tetracycline** QDS for 2 weeks • Treat all sexual contacts	• (As for syphilis)

1 Caused by bacterial infection (continued)

Condition	Site	Description of lesion
Erysipelas	• Face	• Painful, hot, red, swollen patch • Sharply defined edge • Spreads rapidly • Accompanied by swollen glands and fever
Leprosy	• Anywhere	• Anaesthetic skin patches, hypopigmented (for full description, see pages 48–49)
Typhoid	• Anywhere	• A few small pink spots over body following some days of fever (see page 86)

2 Caused by fungal infection

Condition	Site	Description of lesion
Tinea versicolor (Pityriasis)	• Chest (commonly) • Back (commonly) • Face (rarely)	• Macules of different shapes, sizes and colours • Scales come off if lesions scratched
Ringworm		• Papule with thick, red edge and round shape • Dry, white scales in centre of the lesion • Itchy
Candida spp. 'Thrush'	• Mouth • Genitals • Buttocks (in a baby)	• White lesions on mucous membranes of mouth or genitals which are hard to remove, bleeding occurs if they are scraped off • White, itchy vaginal discharge • Red blistered area on buttocks of a baby

3 Caused by parasitic infection

Condition	Site	Description of lesion
Scabies	• Between fingers and toes, round wrists and on elbows, axillae, buttocks, ankles	• Itchy, symmetrical lesions which are papular, vesicular and/or pustular
Tumbu fly abcess	• Anywhere in contact with clothes	• Itchy boil caused by maggot of fly developing (eggs of fly laid on washing hung outside to dry)
Creeping eruptions	• Arms, legs or buttocks	• Itchy, curving line under skin, which moves slowly

Treatment	Prevention
• Hot compresses • Give **Aspirin**, for pain • Give **Penicillin** PO or IM until 2 days after lesions have cleared	
• See pages 48–49	
• Give **Chloramphenicol** (see pages 86–87)	• Cook food properly • Good hygiene

• None needed	
• Wash skin with soap and water • Apply **Benzoic acid** ointment to lesions BD for 10 days *or* 1 g/day **Griseofulvin** for adults ($\frac{1}{2}$ g/day for children)	• Regular washing with soap and water • Prompt treatment
• Give **Nystatin** drops for mouth • Give **Nystatin** tablets or pessaries for vaginal infection • Give **Nystatin** cream for vulva and for buttocks of a baby	

• Soap and water bath, then dry • Use 1 part **Benzyl benzoate** to 3 parts water *or* 1 part **Gamma Benzene hexachloride** to 19 parts water; apply to whole of body, leave, repeat each day for 3 days • Wash clothes, blankets etc. • Treat all members of a family	• Regular washing
• Apply **Vaseline** to the abcess so that maggot emerges and can be removed	• Iron washing
• Crush **Thiabendazole** tablets into vaseline and apply	• Wear shoes

4 Caused by viral infection

Condition	Site	Description of lesion
Chickenpox	• Starts on body, then spreads to faces, arms and legs	• Round red macules → papules → vesicles → pustules. These break open, then crust forms • Itchy + +
Herpes zoster	• As above	• Pain • Lesions like chickenpox but follow the path of nerves • May affect the eye therefore need specialist treatment
Herpes simplex 'Cold sore'	• Lips • Genitals (Herpes simplex Type II)	• Painful red macule → papule → vesicle → pustule; then crusts • Tingling sensation in lesion in early stages • Recurrent and may be associated with poor health, menstruation etc.
Measles	• Starts behind the ears, then spreads all over the body	• Macules and papules • Not itchy (see pages 80-81)
Molluscum contagiosum	• Face, neck, arms, thighs and genitals	• Symmetrical, small, hard, round, solid papules • Multiple

5 Caused by dietary deficiency

Kwashiorkor	• Anywhere	• 'Flaking paint' rash (see pages 88-93)
Pellagra (**Vit B** deficiency)		• Painful, red symmetrical lesions on skin where exposed to sun. Become dark, rough, scaly with well defined edge (see page 91)

6 Caused by allergy

Allergic reaction to: • Food • Drugs • Insect bites • Detergents	• Anywhere	• Pale itchy papules with surrounding redness
Eczema	• Anywhere, but especially arms, elbows, behind knees, neck	• Symmetrical, red, scaly lesions, usually dry but may be wet and weeping in acute phase • Itchy

Other causes of skin lesion
- Cutaneous leishmaniasis ⎫
- African trypanosomiasis ⎬
- American trypanosomiasis ⎬ (see pages 72-77)
- Relapsing fever ⎬
- Typhus ⎭
- Onchocerciasis (see pages 62-63)

Treatment	Prevention
• Apply **Calamine** to itchy lesions • Apply **Gentian Violet** to any infected lesions	
• As above	
• Apply **Gentian Violet** to lesion if septic	
• See pages 80–81	• Immunise
• Scrape with a needle • Apply **Iodine**	

• See pages 88–93	• Good nutrition
• Give **Vit B** tablets TDS till the rash has gone • Improve diet to include meat, eggs, beans, vegetables	• Good nutrition

• Define the cause and take the appropriate action • Apply **Calamine** lotion as necessary • If severe, **Antihistamine** injection (e.g. **Promethazine**) may be needed	
• ? **Calamine** lotion • Try not to scratch • ?**Steroid** ointment • Cold compresses	

Leprosy

Leprosy is estimated to affect 15 million people in the world, only $2\frac{1}{2}$ million have ever been treated (WHO 1980)

Cause and incubation period	Transmission	Diagnosis
Mycobacterium leprae Approximately 10 years	• Nasal secretions • Heavily infected skin ulcer • ? clothing, bedding and utensils contaminated by infected discharges • ? transplacental • ? via breast milk ducts *Reaction to contact with leprosy infection depends on host's immune response — many in contact, few have disease*	• Clinical picture • Slit skin smear from ear lobe or edge of lesion using modified Ziehl-Neelsen stain; look for acid-fast bacilli • Noseblow; stain and examine as above

Classification of leprosy

1 Tuberculoid (TT)   Determinate
2 Borderline Tuberculoid (BT) ⎫
3 Borderline Borderline (BB) ⎬ Indeterminate
4 Borderline Lepromatous (BL) ⎭
5 Lepromatous (LL)   Determinate

Tuberculoid
- High cell-mediated immunity
- Skin lesions
  - few
  - asymmetrical
  - dry
  - anaesthetic
  - saucer right way up
  - sharply demarcated from surrounding skin
  - hypopigmented in dark skin
  - red, erythematous in light skin
- Destruction of hair follicles
- Loss of sweat gland function
- Nerve involvement limited and asymmetrical
- Lepromin test positive

Lepromatous
- Low cell-mediated immunity
- Skin lesions
  - multiple
  - symmetrical
  - greasy
  - not anaesthetic
  - saucer wrong way up
  - ill defined and diffuse
  - hypo/depigmented in dark skin
  - erythematous in light skin
- Thickening of skin
- Coarsening of features
- Ulceration of nasal mucosa and destruction of nasal septum → 'saddlenose'
- Loss of eyebrows and eyelashes
- Nerve trunks thickened (ulnar, median, aural facial, lateral, popliteal)
- Swelling of infected lymph glands
- Testicular atrophy and gynaecomastia
- Lepromin test negative

Treatment
*Resistance to **Dapsone** increasing worldwide, so multiple drug therapy recommended*
- 10 mg/kg **Rifampicin** once a month ⎫
  300 mg **Clofazimine** once a month (in children dose ⎬ administered at leprosy treatment centre
      adapted to body weight) ⎭
  50 mg **Clofazimine** daily or 100 mg on alternate days (adults) ⎫
      100 mg twice a week (children) ⎬ self-administered
  0.9–1.4 mg/kg **Dapsone** daily ⎭

Reactions to treatment (usually)

NB Do *not* suspend treatment

- *Type I reaction: 'upgrading reaction' as cell mediated immunity ↑ and patient going from LL → TT*
    - erythematous, oedematous, warm skin lesions
    - nerve pain, damage and abcesses (may be very rapid damage)

  Rx **Paracetamol**
  Steroids — 0.6-2.0 mg/kg/day **Prednisolone** in divided doses

- *Type II reaction: erythema nodosum leprosum*
    - red, hot, swollen, tender swellings in skin appearing in crops over interval of days
    - arthritis: may be mild to severe
    - iritis
    - neuritis: pain, swelling and loss of function
    - nephritis → albuminuria

  Rx **Mild:**   Bedrest and **Aspirin**
  Moderate: ≤ 300 mg/day **Clofazimine** for up to $\frac{3}{12}$ and **Aspirin**
  Severe: Bedrest; 0.6-2 mg/kg/day **Prednisolone** in divided doses, rapidly reducing to minimum. If this is no help: 100 mg **Thalidomide** QDS (adult)
  NB Do *not* use **Thalidomide** if any possibility of pregnancy, therefore not to women of childbearing age

Type of leprosy depends on the immune response of the patient

If untreated, TT leprosy may deteriorate towards LL leprosy

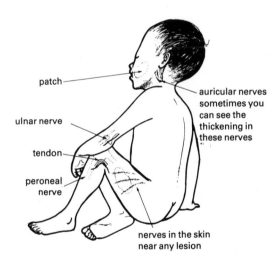

patch

auricular nerves
sometimes you
can see the
thickening in
these nerves

ulnar nerve

tendon

peroneal
nerve

nerves in the skin
near any lesion

Where to look for thickened nerves

For LL and BB leprosy: treat for a minimum of 2 years until skin smear shows no bacilli

For TT leprosy: treat for a minimum of 6 months

- Health education to prevent damage to feet, hands, etc. due to anaesthesia (burns, damage from wrong position of feet, prolonged pressure)
- Provision of shoes; correction of foot drop by splinting
- Eye damage (result of inability to close eye), patient may need tarsorrhaphy
- Correction of damage to instrinsic hand muscles

Diarrhoea

Definition: An abnormal frequency and liquidity of faecal discharge. 6 million children under 5 years old die from it per year.

Cause and incubation period	Aetiology	Diagnosis	Clinical features
Salmonella spp. (including *Salmonella typhi*, i.e. typhoid) Food poisoning 12-48 hours	Food		• Abdominal pain • Fever • Vomiting • Anaemia (in *Salmonella typhi* in children) • Convulsions (in *Salmonella typhi* in children)
Clostridium perfringens 'Pigbel'	Ingestion of pork and a food containing trypsin inhibitor (e.g. sweet potato)		• Paralytic ileus • Abdominal pain
Amoebiasis *Entamoeba histolytica* None	Faeco-oral	• RBCs, amoebae and cysts in stool • WCC ↑ • Hb ↓	• 80% asymptomatic • Bloody diarrhoea with mucus • Fever (if liver abcess) • Liver abcess
Giardiasis *Giardia lamblia*	Faeco-oral: • Cysts on hands • Contaminated water	• Cysts in stool	• No blood in stool • Flatulence • Stools bulky and frothy • Weight loss and anorexia • Malabsorption
Cholera *Vibrio cholerae* 'Classical' 'El Tor' Few hours to 7 days, average 2-3 days	Faeco-oral Large number of symptomless carriers		• Rapid dehydration: up to 5 l/day if no replacement, more if replaced • Hypovolaemic shock • Vomiting • 'Rice water' stools i.e. mucus, odourless • Muscle cramps (due to interstitial fluid loss) • Mental confusion (due to acidosis) • Weakness and heart irregularities (due to potassium loss) • Cyanosis • Acute renal failure • Hypoglycaemia ⎤ • Convulsions ⎟ in • Fever ⎟ children • Paralytic ileus ⎦

Treatment	Prevention
• Rehydration (see page 55) • If *Salmonella typhi* or invasive (i.e. fever > 48 hours, rose spots, splenomegaly) give 50 mg/kg/day **Chloramphenicol** in 4 divided doses until afebrile, then 30 mg/kg/day for 2 weeks	• Cook food properly
• ? surgery to relieve obstruction	
• Give 12-60 mg/kg/day **Metronidazole (Flagyl)** in 3 divided doses for 5 days (400 TDS — adult) and 0.5 g **Diloxanide furoate (Furamide)** TDS for 10 days If severe: add 500 mg **Tetracycline** TDS for 5 days and 65 mg **Emetine hydrochloride** IM daily (adult dose) until diarrhoea subsides	• Sanitation • Safe water • Personal hygiene
• Give **Metronidazole** (as for amoebiasis)	• Sanitation • Safe water • Personal hygiene
• Rapid rehydration to make up entire deficit in 2-4 hours, after giving 1 litre in 10-15 minutes (in severe dehydration, 10% body weight is lost). Use **Ringer's lactate (Hartmann's)** *or* WHO solution, *or* 2 parts **N/saline** to 1 part **Ringer's**. • Maintain hydration via IVI, NG tube or PO to replace loss in stools plus 500 ml • Nurse on 'cholera cot', so that fluid loss can be measured • Give 25 mg/kg/day **Tetracycline** in 4 divided doses for 5 days when vomiting has stopped • General hygiene when nursing patient (barrier nursing not necessary)	• Sanitation • Safe water • Personal hygiene

Diarrhoea (continued)

Cause and incubation period	Aetiology	Diagnosis	Clinical features
Dysentery 'Bacillary dysentery' • *Shigella* spp. • *Campylobacter* • *Balantidium coli*	Faeco-oral		• Blood and mucus in stool • Fever • Abdominal pain • Tenesmus (*Shigella* spp.) • Vomiting (*Shigella* spp. and *Campylobacter*)
Gastroenteritis			• Diarrhoea and vomiting • Abdominal pain • Fever • Signs of dehydration
Measles (in children)	Rash throughout GIT	• Koplik's spots • Rash etc.	• Diarrhoea
Malnutrition Lactase deficiency		• Test for sugar in stool with Clinitest	
Weaning			
Any infection in children			
Schistosomiasis mansoni	Faeco-oral	• Eggs in stool	• Blood in stool • Other symptoms (see page 65)
***Trichuris* sp.** (Whipworm)	Faeco-oral	• Eggs in stool	• Rectal prolapse (in children) • Anaemia
Escherichia coli			
Rotavirus			• Especially in children
Malaria especially *Plasmodium falciparum*			• Especially in adults

Treatment	Prevention
• Rehydration	• Sanitation • Safe water • Personal hygiene
• Rehydrate (antibiotics usually useless)	• As above
• Rehydrate • Maintain hydration and diet	• Vaccinate
• Give lactose-free diet and then gradually reintroduce lactose	
• Rehydrate	
• Treat infection appropriately • Rehydrate	
• Treat schistosomiasis • Rehydrate	• Sanitation • Safe water • Hygiene
• 100 mg **Mebendazole** BD for 3 days • Rehydrate	• Sanitation • Safe water • Hygiene
• Rehydrate	
• Rehydrate	
• Treat malaria (see page 18) • Rehydrate	

Dehydration

Principle of rehydration

That the loss of fluid and electrolytes is the main cause of mortality and morbidity in diarrhoeal disease. Antibiotic treatment is rarely effective except in specific cases.

Assessment of the extent of dehydration

The dehydration score

Where to look	Points to score for the signs you find		
	1	2	3
The whole child (well or 'ill')	'Well'	Restless, irritable, or abnormally quiet, drowsy, or 'floppy'	Delirious, comatose or shocked, very 'ill'
Skin	Normal elasticity	Moderately reduced elasticity	Severely reduced elasticity
Eyes	Normal	Moderately sunken	Severely sunken
Respiration	20-30/min	30-40/min	40-60/min
Mouth	Normal	Dry	Dry and cyanosed
Pulse	Strong, less than 120/min	120-140/min	Over 140/min

If score of:		Give:
6	Mild dehydration (5% body weight lost)	150 ml/kg/dav ORS
6-12	Moderate dehydration (8% body weight lost)	200 ml/kg/day ORS or intraperitoneal if vomiting
13 or more	Severe dehydration	250 ml/kg/day IV or intraperitoneal

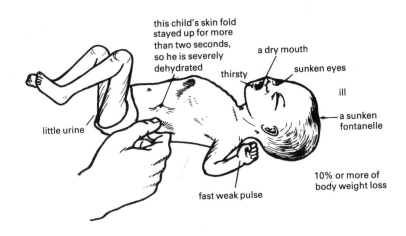

Methods of rehydration

Aim: to replace the water and electrolytes lost in diarrhoea

a) Oral rehydration solution (ORS)

1 litre water
3.5 g salt
2.5 g sodium bicarbonate
1.5 g potassium chloride
20 g glucose (or sugar)

or

1 litre water
$\frac{1}{4}$ teaspoon salt
$\frac{1}{4}$ teaspoon sodium bicarbonate
8 teaspoons sugar

} *or* $\frac{1}{2}$ teaspoon salt

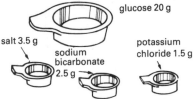

glucose 20 g

salt 3.5 g

sodium bicarbonate 2.5 g

potassium chloride 1.5 g

another spoon to measure salt and sugar is also available from TALC

Measuring scoop (available from TALC)

If no potassium chloride is available, use fresh orange juice
If no glucose or sugar is available, use rice water
Give 2 glasses (of 200 ml) per stool to an adult or $\frac{1}{2}$ –1 glass (of 200 ml) per stool to a child. Give orally, little and often or, in the case of a baby, via nasogastric tube.

b) Intraperitoneal

Use IV solutions (dosage in table opposite). Give over 10 minutes. It is absorbed over 4 hours.

c) Intravenous

Use only if severe dehydration or if other methods are impossible. For a child, use a scalp vein.

Worms (helminths)

SOIL-TRANSMITTED HELMINTHS

Name	Distribution	Appearance and transmission
Ascaris lumbricoides 'Roundworm'	Worldwide 1:4 of the world's population affected	Adult: 25–30 cm Egg: 60 μm *Diagnosis:* • Eggs in stool *Life cycle:* Eggs in faeces → Contaminated soil → 1st, 2nd & 3rd stage larva in egg → Egg ingested → Hatch in GIT → Lymph → Lungs → 4th stage larva → GIT → Eggs in faeces
Trichuris spp. Whipworm	Worldwide	Adult: 4 cm Egg: 55 μm *Diagnosis:* • Eggs in stool • Rectal sigmoidoscope *Life cycle:* Adults in caecum → Eggs in faeces → Faecal contamination of soil → Development to infective larva in soil → Egg swallowed → Hatch → Adults in caecum
Necator americanus and *Ancylostoma* spp. Hookworm	Tropics and subtropics	Adult: 1 cm, hooked head Egg: 60μm *Diagnosis:* • Eggs in stool ++ *Life cycle:* Eggs in faeces → Larvae in soil → Infective larva → Penetrate skin → Blood → Heart → Lungs → GIT → Eggs in faeces
Strongyloides spp.	Worldwide S. America, Africa and Asia	Adult: 2 mm *Life cycle:* Adults → Larvae in faeces → Freeliving larvae → Freeliving adults → soil → 3rd stage larva → Penetrate skin → Adults. Larvae in faeces → soil

Clinical features	Treatment	Prevention
<ul><li>Cough</li><li>GIT disturbance and pain</li><li>Pneumonitis</li><li>Fever</li><li>GIT, bile duct or pancreatic duct obstruction</li></ul>	<ul><li>Give 2.5 mg/kg **Levamisole** stat *or* 75 mg/kg **Piperazine** daily for 2 days *or* 100 mg **Mebendazole** BD for 3 days</li></ul>	<ul><li>Sanitation</li><li>Compost faeces for 1 year before using as fertilizer</li><li>Good personal hygiene</li></ul>
<ul><li>GIT disturbance</li><li>Diarrhoea</li><li>Rectal prolapse } in children</li><li>Anaemia</li></ul>	<ul><li>Give 100 mg **Mebendazole** BD for 3 days (not to children under 2)</li></ul>	<ul><li>Sanitation</li><li>Compost faeces</li><li>Personal hygiene</li></ul>
<ul><li>'Ground itch'</li><li>Cough (larvae in lungs)</li><li>Anaemia</li><li>Bacterial infection at site of penetration—symptoms depend on number of worms, species, iron intake</li></ul>	<ul><li>Replace iron by mouth (**Ferrous sulphate**)</li><li>Give 100 mg **Mebendazole** BD for 3 days (not in pregnancy) *or* 10–20 mg/kg **Pyrantel pamoate** stat</li></ul>	<ul><li>Sanitation</li><li>Compost faeces</li><li>Hygiene</li><li>Wear shoes</li></ul>
<ul><li>'Ground itch'</li><li>Pneumonitis, cough and wheeze</li><li>**Hyperinfection syndrome** If body loses defences against auto infection (e.g. steroids, multiple disease, malnutrition) → septicaemia, encephalitis etc., serous effusions, paralytic ileus, death</li><li>Larva currens (raised, wiggly line on skin of trunk, itchy, appears in crops, comes and goes within few hours)</li></ul>	<ul><li>Give 25 mg/kg **Thiabendazole** BD for 3 days</li></ul>	<ul><li>Very difficult</li></ul>

Worms (helminths) (continued)

Name	Distribution	Appearance and transmission
Toxocara canis Visceral larva migrans	Worldwide	*Diagnosis:* • Difficult Dog → Eggs in faeces → Eggs ingested from soil or fur → Hatch → Adults
Trichinella spp.	Worldwide	Adult: < 3 mm *Life cycle:* Adults in GIT of pig or rat → Larval stage in muscles → Meat not cooked properly → Eaten by next host → Adults in GIT → Larva in muscles
Enterobius sp. Threadworm	Worldwide	Adult: 1 cm Egg: 55 μm *Life cycle:* Adults in caecum → Female to anus → Eggs on skin of anus → Larva in egg → Egg swallowed → Adults in caecum
Taenia solium (Pig tapeworm) *Taenia saginata* (Beef tapeworm)	Worldwide	Adult: *T. saginata* 3–10 m *T. solium* 2–7 m Egg: 36–40 μm *Life cycle:* Cyst swallowed in meat → Adult in GIT (man) → Eggs in faeces → Swallowed → GIT → Blood → Muscles → Encyst → Cyst swallowed in meat
Echinococcus spp. Hydatid disease (Tapeworm)	Worldwide	Adult: 3–9 mm *Life cycle:* Carnivore: worm in GIT → Eggs in faeces → Cyst in herbivore (or man) → Infected meat eaten → Carnivore: worm in GIT

TAPEWORMS

Clinical features	Treatment	Prevention
• Fever • Eosinophilia • Hepatomegaly • Asthma • Eye granuloma	• Give **Thiabendazole** over prolonged period	• Difficult • Regular deworming of dogs
• Muscle damage and pain • GIT disturbance • Fever • Oedema round eyes		• Cook meat thoroughly • Freeze meat for 20 days
• Itching • Appendicitis	• Apply **Thiabendazole** paste around the anus — to make the paste crush **Thiabendazole** tablets in soft white Paraffin/ Vaseline	
• Abdominal pain • Loss of weight • Anorexia • Muscle cysts • Cysts in CNS	For *T. solium* and *T. saginata* • Give 50 mg/kg/day **Niclosamide** as 2 doses one hour apart	• Effective sanitation • Proper cooking of meat • Inspection of meat • Freeze meat for $\frac{10}{365}$

• Cysts
  — 70% in liver → hepatomegaly
  — 20% in lungs → cough and dyspnoea
  — 10% elsewhere
    brain → signs of tumour *or*
    bone → pain
• Anaphylactic shock due to rupture of cyst
	• Surgery: cyst must be removed *intact*. If not possible, inject cyst with 10-20 ml 10% **Formalin** after withdrawing 10-20 ml of cyst fluid	• Hygiene
		• Deworming of dogs
		• Do not allow dogs to eat infected meat (e.g. dead sheep)

Worms (helminths) (continued)

Name (Habitat of adult)	Distribution	Appearance and transmission
Fasciolopis sp. (GIT)	Far East, India	Adult: 2–7 cm Egg: 120 μm *Fasciola* spp. (Liver) — Worldwide *Diagnosis*: eggs in stool *Life cycle:* Man, Pig, Sheep → Eggs in faeces → Contaminated water → Snails → Vegetation → Vegetation eaten (wild watercress) → Man, Pig, Sheep Pig — *Fasciolopis* Sheep — *Fasciola*
Opisthorchis spp. (Liver) *Clonorchis* sp. (Liver) *Heterophyes* sp. (GIT) *Metagonimus* sp. (GIT)	Middle and Far East	Adult : 5 mm–2 cm Attached to GIT wall or bile duct Egg: 30 μm *Diagnosis*: eggs in stool *Life cycle:* Man → Eggs in faeces → Contaminated water → Snail → Encyst in fish → Fish eaten → Man
Paragonimus spp. (Lung)	Far East, India, W. Africa	Adults: like coffee bean Egg: 90 μm × 60 μm *Diagnosis*: eggs in stool or sputum *Life cycle:* Man → Eggs in faeces → Contaminated water → Snail → Crabs and crayfish → Eaten → Man
Guinea worm *Dracunculus medinensis*	Africa, Middle East, USSR, Indian subcontinent	Adult: ♀ 1 m long ♂ 25 mm *Incubation period*: 12 months Especially prevalent at end of dry season *Life cycle:* Larva from ulcer → Water → Cyclops (water flea) → 12 days → Ingested by man → Larva from ulcer

(For Schistosomes, i.e. blood flukes, see page 64)

FLUKES

FILARIAL WORM

Clinical features	Treatment	Prevention
• Ascites • Local GIT ulceration • Diarrhoea • Intestinal obstruction • Toxaemia → death *Fasciola* spp. (Liver) • Adults in bile ducts → haemobilia • Intermittent obstructive jaundice • Eosinophilia	• Give 0.1ml/kg **Tetrachlorethylene** PO *or* 0.25 g/kg/day **Bephenium hydrochloride** for 3 days • Give 30 mg/kg' **Praziquantel** BD for 3 days	• Not using night soil (faeces) as fertilizer • Compost • Not eating water vegetation • Proper cooking of food
Opisthorchis spp. and *Clonorchis* sp. • Obstructive jaundice • Fever • Feeling of something in liver *Heterophyes* sp. and *Metagonimus* sp. • As for *Fasciolopsis* sp.	• Give 30 mg/kg **Praziquantel** BD for 3 days • As for *Fasciolopsis* sp.	• Not using faeces as fertilizer • Composting • Sanitation • Cooking food
• Cough and haemoptysis • Cysts in lungs • Cysts in other tissues • Cavitation and fibrosis of lungs	• Give 20 mg/kg **Praziquantel** BD for 3 days	• Sanitation • Not using faeces as fertilizer • Cooking fish etc.
Just before worm discharges larvae: • Urticaria and blister • Periorbital oedema • Wheezing • Fever • Vomiting? • Local sepsis • Local or general allergy • Rarely, in CNS → paraplegia	• Dressings • Antibiotics PRN • Gradual extraction • Filter water	• Protect water supplies e.g. walls round wells • Use **Abate** insecticide for drinking water • Filter water

Worms (helminths) (continued)

Name	Distribution	Diagnosis	Transmission
Wuchereria bancrofti	Tropical Africa, Asia (S.E. Pacific), N of S. America	• Filter several ml blood to see microfilariae in blood	Infected man → Microfilariae sucked up by biting insects → Develop to 3rd stage larva → Infective larvae migrate to proboscis → Penetrate when insect feeds → Infected man
Brugia malayi	Indonesia and S.E. Asia, S. India		

Filarial worm		Vector
W. bancrofti	—	*Aedes* and *Culex* mosquitos
B. malayi	—	*Anopheles* and *Mansonia* mosquitos
Loa Loa	—	*Chrysops* fly
T. perstans	—	*Culicoides* midge
T. streptocerca	—	*Culicoides* midge
M. ozzardi	—	*Culicoides* midge *Simulium* blackfly
O. volvulus	—	*Simulium* blackfly (breeds in fast flowing rivers)

Name	Distribution	Diagnosis
Loa loa	Rain forest of W. and C. Africa	• Microfilariae found in blood from an earlobe between 10 am and 2 pm (Giemsa stain)
Tetrapetalonema perstans	Forests of Ghana, Zaire and Cameroon	• Microfilariae found in blood
Tetrapetalonema streptocerca	Forests of Ghana, Zaire and Cameroon	
Manzonella ozzardi	W. Indies, N and C of S. America	
Onchocerca volvulus Onchocerciasis 'River blindness'	Forest and savannah of tropical Africa, N of S. America, Yemen	• Put skin snips from calf, thigh, hip, or iliac crest into saline and look for microfilariae after 2-3 hours

Clinical features	Treatment	Prevention
Depends on species, number of worms, length of infection, host immunity • Recurrent fever • Painful lymphadenopathy leading to damage, thickening and blockage — lymphoedema — hydrocele — elephantiasis — chyluria • Tropical eosinophilia	• Give 2–3 mg/kg **Diethylcarbamazine (DEC)** TDS for $\frac{21}{365}$ after Day 1 50 mg stat Day 2 50 mg BD Day 3 50 mg TDS (for adults) i.e. treatment should be started on a small dose and gradually increased • Supportive bandaging • Surgery for scrotum and hydrocele	• Control mosquitoes • Use repellents • Prompt treatment
• Calabar swellings which are painful and itchy in SC tissues, they subside in days • Worm in the eye causes irritation swelling and pain • Eosinophilia	• **DEC** (as above) • Surgical extraction of worms	• Regular chemotherapy with 200 mg **DEC** TDS for 3 days per month
• Non pathogenic		
• Allergic skin reaction	• **DEC**	
• Onchocermata which are SC nodules containing adults, especially in pelvis and chest • Intense skin irritation • Hyperpigmentation of skin called 'leopard skin' • Skin thin and wrinkled • Hanging groin • Iritis, sclerosing keratitis, inflammation of choroid and retina, optic nerve damage → blindness	• Use **DEC** to kill microfilariae Day 1 50 mg Day 2 100 mg Day 3 200 mg Day 4 200 mg BD Day 5 ⎫ Day 6 ⎬ 200 mg TDS Day 7 ⎭ (adults) Mazzotti reaction — papular dermatitis, adenopathy, postural hypotension, precipitation of iritis Rx **Steroids** • 100 mg **Suramin** (adults)	• Insecticides in rivers **(Abate)** • Decrease flow of rivers • Siting of housing away from waterways and endemic areas • Protective clothing

Schistosomiasis

Schistosomiasis affects approximately 100 million people in the world

Type and distribution	Transmission	Pathology
Schistosoma japonicum Far East, S.E. Asia	See below	Larva → Skin → Blood → Develop into adults → Adults lie paired in blood vessels and block venules of liver or bladder (sexual reproduction) → Eggs enter tissues → Inflammation and fibrosis → Passed out in stools or urine → Contaminate water → Infect snails → Asexual reproduction → (Larva)
Schistosoma mansoni Africa, America, M. East		
Schistosoma haematobium Africa, M. East		

child spreading infection

schistosome eggs being passed in the urine

snail

child being infected

egg

second kind of larva (cercaria) coming out of snail and going into child

schistosomes multiplying inside snail (asexual reproduction)

larva swimming (miracidium)

How Schistosoma haematobium is spread

Diagnosis	Clinical features	Treatment	Prevention
• Eggs in stool (concentrated) (1500 eggs are produced each day)	• 'Swimmers itch' at the site of penetration • Circumoval granuloma → fibrosis • 'Katayama fever' (1st sign) — fever — urticaria — eosinophilia • Diarrhoea with blood • Hepatomegaly • Splenomegaly • Cough and wheeze • Cachexia • Lethargy • Oesophageal varices • CNS compression (*S. japonicum* only) • 'Cerebral tumour' signs (*S. japonicum* only)	• 25 mg/kg/day **Niradazole (Ambilhar)** PO in 3 divided doses for 5–10 days S/E GIT disturbance and/or psychosis therefore given under supervision in hospital *or* 40 mg/kg **Praziquantel** PO (expensive) as single dose	• Sanitation • Killing of snails with molluscicide • Chemotherapy to known disease cases and to local population on regular basis • Discourage swimming etc. in infested water (Irrigation schemes may increase the incidence of schistosomiasis)
• Eggs in stool (concentrated) (300 eggs are produced each day)	• As above *and* • Oesophageal varices • Portal hypertension	As for *S. japonicum*	
• Eggs in urine specimen (between 12 pm and 2 pm)	• 'Swimmers itch' • 'Katayama fever' • Splenomegaly • Cough and wheeze • Haematuria (terminal) • Pseudopapillomas of bladder • Hydroureter and hydronephrosis • Nephrotic syndrome	• 10 mg/kg **Metrifonate** PO on days 0, 14 and 28	

Liver diseases

Disease and incubation period	Aetiology	Clinical features
Viral hepatitis **Type A** 15–45 days **Type B** 30–150 days **Non A, non B** 15-150 days	• Faeco-oral • In all body fluids: faeces; blood; semen; etc. • By bedbugs • As for type B	Often asymptomatic, but otherwise • Anorexia • Malaise • Fever • Jaundice (less in Type A) • Vomiting • Tender hepatomegaly • Urticaria (Type B) • In 5% cases of Type B → acute liver failure • In pregnancy it is dangerous → acute hepatic necrosis and chronic disease and can be transmitted to a baby at birth • Dark urine and pale stools • Aches and pains • Upper abdominal discomfort
Liver cirrhosis	• Viral hepatitis • Alcohol • Toxins • Iron poisoning	
Acute liver failure	Hepatitis B	• Flapping tremor • ↓ consciousness • Haemorrhage • Hypoglycaemia
Hepatoma (high incidence in developing countries)	• Viral hepatitis • Aflatoxin	• Abdominal pain • Ascites • Hard irregular hepatomegaly • Jaundice • Wasting
Amoebic liver abcess	Amoeba → liver via portal vein → abcess May rupture into • Peritoneum • Pleural cavity • Pericardium • Through skin *Diagnosis:* amoebae or cysts in stool	• Enlarged, tender liver • Cough or breathlessness, if lung involved • Anaemia • Jaundice (10%) • Localised oedema and tenderness of skin over abcess • Cutaneous sinus • Abcess with 'anchovy sauce' pus • Fever • Inflammation of area into which abcess ruptures

Some other diseases affecting the liver in tropical countries

• Leptospirosis
• Clonorchiasis (see page 60)
• Yellow fever

• AIDS (see page 70)
• Malaria (see page 16)
• Kwashiorkor (see page 90)

Treatment	Prevention
• Little available except rest	• Improve sanitation • No unnecessary injections • Screen blood for blood transfusions • Gammaglobulin to contacts of hepatitis Type A to give $\frac{3}{12}$ protection • Vaccine to those at risk of hepatitis Type B 10-12 μg on day 0, 28 and $\frac{6}{12}$; lasts 5 years (but expensive)
• Stop alcohol • Use diuretics • Give transfusion	
• Give **Glucose** IV • Restrict protein • Give **Neomycin** • ?haemodialysis 20% will recover	
• Give analgesics • TLC	• Prevent hepatitis Type B by vaccination • Proper storage of grain and legumes to prevent aflatoxin development
• Give 50 mg/kg/day **Metronidazole (Flagyl)** in 3 divided doses for 7 days *and* • 0.5 g **Diloxanide furoate (Furamide)** TDS for 5-10 days	• Sanitation • Safe water • Personal hygiene

• Hydatid cysts (see page 58)
• Relapsing fever (see page 76)
• Sickle-cell disease (see page 20)
• Leishmaniasis (see page 74)

• Chronic infection (e.g. TB)
• Poisoning with bush teas (W. Indies, M. East and Africa)

Sexually transmitted diseases

↑ *incidence with:*
- ↑ number of sexual contacts
- ↑ use of alcohol
- ↑ asymptomatic carriers
- ↑ travel
- ↑ resistance to Penicillin
- ↑ homosexuality
- ↑ use of 'Pill' and intra-uterine device rather than sheaths

Disease and cause	Incubation period	Pathology	Diagnosis
Gonorrhoea *Gonococcus*	3–10 days	• Symptoms only last for a short while, but the disease will continue to affect patient → long term problems • Dangerous if a baby is born to a mother with gonorrhoea → gonococcal ophthalmitis which needs intensive eye treatment to prevent blindness	• Urethral, cervical or vaginal smear
Syphilis *Treponema pallidum*	3 weeks (9–90 days)	• Very common disease If untreated, organism stays in body and enters blood and cerebro-spinal fluid → long term effects	• Microscopy of chancre • Serological tests
Lympho-granuloma venereum *Chlamydia*		• More common in developing countries than in the West	• Clinical picture

Clinical features	Treatment	Prevention
• Urethral discharge • Dysuria and frequency • Lower abdominal pain (♀) • Slight vaginal discharge • 50% of women are asymptomatic *After months or years:* • Amenorrhoea • Sterility • Joint swelling and pain (♂)	• Give 4 megaunits **Procaine Penicillin** IM and 1g **Probenecid** PO *or* 5 megaunits **Crystalline Penicillin** and 1g **Probenecid** PO *or* 2g **Ampicillin** PO and 1 g **Probenecid** • Treat all sexual contacts • Follow up for 3 weeks	• Avoid indiscriminate sex • Treat all disease promptly • Use of sheaths • Health education

1° • Chancre (sore) on genitalia, lips or anus it will heal in 3–8 weeks
  • Lymphadenopathy
2° • **Lasts 3–12 months**
  • Serology positive
  • Non-itchy skin rash
  • Malaise
  • Headache and fever
  • Sore throat
  • Lymphadenopathy
  • Swollen joints
3° • **2–10 years later**
  • Chronic ulcers (gumma) of skin, bone and liver
  • Neurosyphilis
  • Insanity
  • Aortic valvular disease of heart and/or aortic aneurysm
  • Death
	• Give 600 000–1 million units **Procaine Penicillin** per day IM for 10–14 days
	or, if allergic to Penicillin, 750 mg **Tetracycline** QDS for 10 days *or* 500 mg **Erythromycin** QDS
	• Give serological tests to make sure that the disease is cured, check for up to 2 years
	• Trace and treat all sexual contacts
		• As for gonorrhoea

• Small genital ulcer • Swelling and ulceration of local lymph glands • Fever • Genital elephantiasis • Vescico-vaginal fistula • Rectal stricture (homosexual male)	• 250–500 mg **Tetracycline** QDS for 2 weeks • Treat all sexual contacts	• As for gonorrhoea

Sexually transmitted diseases (continued)

Disease and cause	Incubation period	Pathology	Diagnosis
Non-specific urethritis *Chlamydia*	Long		• Urethral or vaginal smear
Genital herpes *Herpes simplex*		• Recurrent virus which lies dormant in between acute episodes • Great risk to baby born vaginally while mother has acute episode, it will need elective LSCS	• Clinical picture
Granuloma inguinale *Donovania granulomatis*			• Biopsy of lesion by scraping and microscopy
Viral hepatitis especially Hepatitis B			
AIDS (Acquired Immuno Deficiency Syndrome)		• Particularly affects homo-sexual population in the West, but endemic in parts of Africa amongst heterosexuals	• Clinical features
Trichomonas vaginalis		• Often occurs in association with gonorrhoea	• High vaginal swab, then microscopy and culture
Candidiasis 'Thrush'	See page 44		

Some other infections which can be transmitted by sexual contact

- Scabies
- Pubic lice
- Amoebiasis
- Giardiasis
- Genital warts
- Genital molluscum contagiosum

Clinical features	Treatment	Prevention
• Urethral discharge • Dysuria • Prostatitis in ♂ • Salpingitis and pelvic inflammatory disease ♀ • Conjunctivitis in babies	• Give 250–500 mg **Tetracycline** QDS for 2 weeks *or* • 500 mg **Erythromycin** QDS	• As for gonorrhoea
• Sores and ulceration of genitalia • ? link with cancer of cervix	• Use **Gentian Violet** *or*, if available, • **Idoxyduridine** ointment • **Acyclovir** is a new drug for this, but *very* expensive.	• As for gonorrhoea
• Chronic ulceration of genitalia	• Give 250 mg **Tetracycline** QDS for 7–14 days (or **Streptomycin**)	• As for gonorrhoea
• Vaginal discharge • Urethritis in ♂	• None available	• As for gonorrhoea
• Kaposi's sarcoma • Lymphomas • Immune deficiency → repeated infections • Anorexia • Lymphadenopathy • Prolonged fever • Weight loss • Death within 1 year	• None available	• As for gonorrhoea
• Profuse yellow/green frothy vaginal discharge with stale, offensive odour • Soreness of genitals • Frequency of micturation and dysuria • Dyspareunia (painful intercourse)	• 200 mg **Metronidazole (Flagyl)** TDS for 7–10 days (not in early pregnancy) • 5 mg **Pentrane** or **Clotrimazole** • Hygiene • Treat all sexual contacts • Exclude gonorrhoea	• As for gonorrhoea

Less common tropical diseases

Disease and incubation period	Distribution	Transmission	Diagnosis
Trypanosomiasis			
African trypanosomiasis 'Sleeping sickness' *Trypanosoma gambiense* from 10 days to months or years Sub-acute or chronic *Trypanosoma rhodesiense* Rapid → death in weeks (20–50 days)	W. and C. Africa as far north as Sudan and as far south as Zaire (usually)	Bite of tsetse fly (*Glossina* sp.) → chancre on skin → trypanosomes in blood → fly bites and is infected → development in fly → fly bites next host Those living near habitat of tsetse fly are most at risk *T. gambiense is a disease of:* • Farmers • Ferrymen • Road/rail builders • Tin miners Reservoir in pigs *T. rhodesiense is a disease of:* • Hunters • Pastoralists • Honey-gatherers Reservoir in game	• Gland aspiration • Thick blood film and look for trypanosomes • Lumbar puncture ↑ cells ↑ protein • ↑ ESR to ≥ 50–100 mm/hr
American trypanosomiasis 'Chaga's disease'	C. and S. America	Triatomine (reduviid) bugs live in walls of houses and feed on people. They deposit faeces, which are scratched into the skin or into the conjunctiva, or ingested → trypanosomes in bloodstream → bug bites infected human → infected → bites next host.	• Thick blood film shows trypanosomes in blood • Serological tests • Amastigotes are in muscle biopsy • Xenodiagnosis, if available

Clinical features	Treatment	Prevention

T. gambiense
1 Chancre which is itchy
2 Systematic invasion
  • Irregular fever
  • Lymphadenopathy —
    'Winterbottom's sign'
  • Hepatosplenomegaly
  • Rashes
  • Puffy oedematous
    swelling of face or body
  • Hyperaesthesia of nerves
3 CNS invasion
  • Headache
  • Personality change
  • Sleepy in the day
  • Delusions and psychoses
  • Backache
  • Chorea or othetosis
  • Consciousness ↓
  • Wasting
 	
T. rhodesiense
  • Myocarditis → heart failure
  • Jaundice
  • Early CNS invasion
  • Lympadenopathy
  • Anaemia
	• *T. gambiense*
	Early stages:
	3–4 mg/kg/day
	Pentamidine IM 7–10
	doses, either daily or on
	alternate days
	• *T. rhodesiense*
	Early stages:
	20mg/kg **Suramin** IV
	on days 1, 3, 7, 14 and
	21 S/E fever, anorexia,
	wasting, exfoliative
	dermatitis
	• *T. rhodesiense* and
	T. gambiense
	CNS involvement:
	0.1 ml/kg **Melarsoprol**
	(Mel B) to maximum
	single dose of 5 ml IV,
	i.e. 3.6 mg/kg/day Re-
	peated courses of 3.6 mg/
	kg/day for 3–4 days, then
	rest for $\frac{7}{365}$ then repeat
	for total of 3 or 4
	courses
	S/E encephalopathy
		• Protective clothing
		• Repellants
		• Insecticides sprayed on
		  vegetation
		• Clearing of vegetation
		  cover
		• Reduce wild game
		• Reduce settlements in
		  endemic areas
		• Early Rx of cases
		• For *T. gambiense* give
		  3–4 mg/kg
		  Pentamidine IM
		  every $\frac{3}{12} - \frac{6}{12}$

Initial infection
• Chancre (chagoma) —
  cutaneous oedema on skin
  or orbital oedema (Romana's
  sign)
Years after initial infection
• Invasion of muscle and
  nerve fibres:
  — heart → cardiac failure
  — CNS → meningo-
    encephalitis
  — GIT → megacolon,
    dysphagia
• Hepatosplenomegaly
• Lymphadenopathy
• Fever
	• Not very effective
	Nifurtimox may help to
	stop parasitemia but will
	not kill intracellular
	parasites
		• Improved housing
		• Insecticides
		  (temporary)

Disease and incubation period	Distribution	Transmission	Diagnosis
Leishmaniasis *1 Visceral* 'Kala-azar' *Leishmania donovani* *Leishmania infantum* (children) 3–18 months (occasionally as short as $\frac{2}{52}$)	Mediterranean, Africa, S. America, C. and E. Asia, India	*Vector:* • Sandflies of genus *Phlebotomus* or *Lutzomyia* *Mammalian hosts:* • Rodents • Sloths (S. America) • Dogs • Jackals • Man infected mammalian host sandfly bites → amastigotes multiply in sandfly promastigates passed on when sandfly bites the next person multiply in 2nd mammalian host	• Amastigotes in — spleen smear — bone marrow — buffy coat • Culture of blood • ↑↑ ESR • Serological tests
2 Cutaneous 'Oriental sore' *Leishmania tropica* *Leishmania mexicana* 2–8 weeks	Mediterranean, Tropical Africa, India	skin nodule phagocytic cells reticulo-endothelial system	• Slit skin smear from edge of ulcer to see amastigotes • Leishmanin skin test positive after cure
3 Muco-cutaneous 'Espundia' *Leishmania braziliensis* 2–8 weeks	S. America	Sandflies breed in dark, moist places (e.g. cracks in walls, caves, anthills, latrines). Bite at dawn, dusk and at night.	• Amastigotes in slit skin smear from early lesion • Leishmanin skin test positive after cure • Serological tests

Clinical features	Treatment	Prevention
• Skin nodule — leishmanoma • High fever • Progressive splenomegaly • Some hepatomegaly • Generalised lymphadenopathy • Weight loss • Greyish pigmentation of skin • Marked anaemia and leucopenia • High serum gamma globulins especially Ig G • Low platelets → bruising and bleeding, especially of the gums • Death within 2 yrs if no Rx *Post Kala-azar dermal leishmaniasis* Occurs after treatment and usually provides a reservoir of infection • Localised or widespread macular or nodular skin eruption	• Give 0.1–0.2 ml/kg/day **Pentavalent Antimony-Sodium stibogluconate** IV or IM for 30 days • The patient should rest • Follow up for ≥ 1 year with repeat cultures and blood tests	• Residual house spraying with insecticide • Catch and destroy stray dogs • Prompt treatment of cases • Sleep on 1st floor of house or on the roof • Separate housing areas from forests by a wide zone cleared of trees (S. America)
• Itchy papule on arms, legs or face → nodule → ulcer with rolled, undermined edge and crust → depressed scar and immunity • Rarely there are diffuse nodules and ulcerated lesions • Lupoid leishmaniasis, looking like skin TB	If one only it will heal spontaneously If multiple: • **Sodium stibogluconate** (as above) • Heat locally • Protection from secondary infection	
• Primary cutaneous sore *Then 1-2 years later:* • Mucosa of nose, mouth and pharynx ulcerated and destroyed • Destruction of tissue and bone	Not satisfactory • **Sodium stibogluconate** (as above) and 250 µg/kg/day **Amphotericin B** increasing to 1 mg/kg/day given daily by IV infusion diluted in 1 litre of 5% **Dextrose**, over 6 h, (and **Nifurtimox**) • **Metronidazole** may prevent 2° anaerobic infection	

Less common tropical diseases (continued)

Disease and incubation period	Distribution	Transmission	Diagnosis
Rickettsiosis *1 Louse-borne typhus* Rickettsia prowazeki 13 days	Ethiopia, Rwanda, Burundi (Worldwide)	Faeces of body lo se scratched into skin and reproduce in lining cells of small blood vessels	• Clinical picture
2 Flea-borne typhus Rickettsia prowazeki var. *mooseri* 13 days	Urban areas, Worldwide	Faeces of flea scratched into skin	• Clinical picture
3 Tick-borne typhus Rickettsia conori 5-7 days	S. and N. Africa, India, Australasia, Siberia, Mediterranean	Infection through bite of hard (ixodid) tick	• Clinical picture
4 Scrub typhus Rickettsia tsutsugam-ushi 12 days	Asia, Australasia	Through bite of chigger mite (found near banana and tree plantations and banks of rivers)	• Clinical picture • Neutropenia
Relapsing fever *1 Louse-borne* Borrelia recurrentis	Worldwide where squalor	Faeces of body louse scratched into skin	• Thick blood film organisms seen after Romanowsky staining
2 Tick-borne Borrelia duttoni	Africa, S. Europe, Middle East, Asia, N., S. and C. America	By bite or by faeces scratched into skin of soft tick (*Ornithodorus* sp.)	

Clinical features	Treatment	Prevention
• High fever for $\frac{2}{52}$ • Severe headache • General aches and pains • Conjunctivitis • Mental dullness • Skin rash • Petechial haemorrhage *R. Mooseri* is milder If no **Rx**: • Pneumonitis • Parotitis • Gangrene • Death *Recurrence:* Brill-Zinsser disease but milder	• Give 25–50 mg/kg/day **Tetracycline** in 4 divided doses for 5–7 days	• Improve hygiene and washing of clothes • Improve social conditions
• High fever for 7 days • General aches and pains • Conjunctivitis • 'Tache noir' ulcer at bite site • Rash after 5 days • Mortailty low	• As above	
• Sudden high fever for 10–14 days • Rash after $\frac{1}{52}$ on palms/soles • Slowness and dullness • Cranial nerve involvement → deafness → squint • Lymph/hepato/splenomegaly (sometimes) • Conjunctivitis • Myocarditis/encephalitis/ pneumonitis	• As above	
• Fever • Headache } for 4–7 days • Prostration • Aches and pains *May remit spontaneously, followed by relapses:* a) 2–3 times in louse-borne relapsing fever b) 3–6 times in tick-borne relapsing fever c) ≤ 11 times in African infections • Myocarditis • Meningo-encephalitis • Lymph/hepato/splenomegaly • Haemorrhagic rash (severe louse-borne relapsing fever) • Liver failure (louse-borne relapsing fever)	• **Tetracycline** (as above) + oral **Corticosteroid** for a few days • **Tetracycline** (as above)	• Mass delousing using powder • Use of sleeping net • Sleep off the floor • Protective clothing • Repellants • Residual spraying to eliminate ticks **(DDT)**

Less common tropical diseases (continued)

Disease and incubation period	Distribution	Transmission	Diagnosis

Rabies
(Rhabdovirus)
	Worldwide except Australia, UK, Hawaii, Scandinavia	In saliva of infected animal
		• Dog
		• Wolf
		• Jackel
		• Fox
		• Squirrel
		• Bat
		• Cat
		Enters via
		• Bite
		• Mucous membrane
		• Skin abrasion
		• Inhalation
			• Clinical picture
			• History
			• Suspect animal if
			  — odd behaviour
			  — unpredictable attack
			  — dysphagia
			  — salivation
			  — senseless biting
			  — pawing mouth
			  — odd barking
			  — paralysis
			• Observe for $\frac{10}{365}$
			  — if dies send for histology
			  — if patient does not die, it is *not* rabies
			• If animal is well 5 days after biting human, it was not infective at the time it bit the human

Mode of infection	Clinical features	Treatment	Prevention
• Virus ascends to CNS and causes meningo-encephalitis • Proliferates in nerve cells in brain and peripheral ganglia	1 'Furious' rabies Rapid onset of: • Pyrexia • Anxiety and terror • Insomnia • Numbness, itching and pain at site of bite • Spasms of pharynx and larynx when tries to swallow → hydrophobia • Spasm of respiratory muscles → aerophobia • Salivation + + + • Paralysis • Death in ≤ 6 days 2 'Dumb' rabies (Rare in man common in dogs and usual in herbivores) • Pyrexia • Malaise • Numbness, itching and pain at site of bite • Numbness • Weakness • Paralysis • Death in approximately 2 weeks	If ill already — none except • **Heroin** • **Chlorprom-azine** • **Amylobarbi-tone** • Barrier nursing with gloves, mask and goggles • TLC	Before bite or after if no sign of illness 1 Treatment of animal bites • Clean wound with 20% salt soap solution, rinse off soap and apply **Quaternary Ammonium compound** • Sterilise penetrating wounds with **Nitric acid** • Remove damaged tissue • Do not suture wound • Vaccinate patient; a long incubation period gives time to build up antibodies. If it is likely to be a short incubation period, give hyper-immune serum 2 Eradicate stray dogs 3 Vaccination • Prophylaxis: give 0.1 ml **Merieux** vaccine intradermally on days 0, 28 and at 6 months: it lasts 3 years • After a bite: give 0.2 ml **Merieux** vaccine in 4 different sites at the same time intradermally (confers immunity in 7 days) (Semple vaccine causes post-vaccinal encephalitis in 1:250 vaccinees)

Infectious diseases and immunisation

'In the less well-developed countries child development and health is dominated by the twin problems of nutritional deficiency and infectious diseases.' (Morley)

Of every 1000 births in developing countries:
- 5 are crippled by polio
- 10 die from neonatal tetanus
- 20 die from whooping cough
- 30 die from measles

Disease and incubation period	General notes	Pathology and aetiology	Diagnosis
Measles 7–14 days If going to isolate infected person, it needs to be until 5 days after the rash has appeared	<ul><li>Mortality in developing countries is 400 × higher than in industrialised countries</li><li>It has the most severe effects on nutrition of all infections</li><li>Some passive immunity at birth — this lasts for 6 months</li><li>Criteria for admission to hospital: — hoarseness, especially if there is laryngeal obstruction — dehydration; blood and mucus in stool or > 5 stools per day — convulsion or loss of consciousness — underweight, especially if < 10th centile — soreness of mouth, especially if interferes with suckling — dyspnoea, especially if flaring of nostrils and ↑ respiratory rate</li></ul>	Droplet infection	<ul><li>Koplik's spots</li><li>Clinical picture</li></ul>

The interaction of malnutrition and infection (from Morley & Woodland 1979)

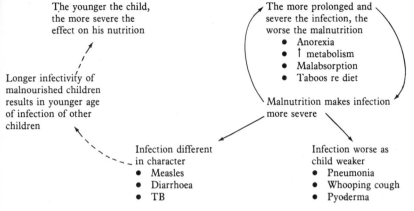

Clinical features	Treatment	Prevention
1 In well-nourished child • Cough and cold for a few days → ? pneumonia • Fever • Rash behind ears, then spreading all over body, disappearing after about 5 days • Koplik's spots in mouth and conjunctiva • Red, watery eyes and photophobia *2 In malnourished child* As above and • Bad rash with desquamation; papules palpable on skin • Severe diarrhoea 2° to enteritis • Pneumonia and other pulmonary problems • Severe eye complications associated with Vit A deficiency • Stomatitis and ulceration of mouth → anorexia 　　　→ predisposition to cancrum oris • Laryngitis • Encephalitis → brain damage and fits • Activation of 1° TB lesion • Precipitates malnutrition in an undernourished child	• Maintain (or correct) hydration • Ensure good nutrition • Give 100 000 IU **Vit A** stat if child malnourished by IM injection stat, and repeat orally on 2nd day (give half dose to child < 1 year) • Keep eyes clean 　— local **Tetracycline** or **Chloramphenicol** ointment 　— If signs of damage give **Atropine** drops to rest eye 　— cover eye PRN to avoid 2° infection • Keep mouth clean and comfortable • Treat fever • If bronchopneumonia, give 50–200 mg/kg/day **Ampicillin** *or* 50–100 mg/kg/day **Chloramphenicol** injection IM If poor response, consider TB; do CXR and change treatment PRN • If laryngitis, give 　— adequate hydration 　— ?humidification 　— ?steroids 　— tracheostomy, if necessary • Encourage breast-feeding for at least $\frac{2}{12}$ after episode of measles	• Measles vaccination (for details, see later) • Improve nutrition • Improve socio-economic conditions (e.g. overcrowding)

Infectious diseases and immunisation (continued)

Disease and incubation period	General notes	Pathology and aetiology	Diagnosis
Whooping cough (Pertussis) 6–18 days	• No passive immunity at birth • Almost all non-immunised children will get whooping cough • If a child gets whooping cough in the 1st year of life → 40% mortaliy • Rarely fatal after 1st year, but complications occur • May relapse for ≤ 1–2 years	• Caused by *Bordatella pertussis* • Droplet infection • Sticky mucus in bronchi → cough before inspiration therefore anoxic before start coughing • Blockage of bronchioles → collapse, obstructive emphysema, pneumothorax • 2° bacterial infection common	Difficult, as culture only positive for 4 weeks
Diphtheria 2–6 days	• Severity depends on virulence of toxin, amount of toxin absorbed and extent of membrane • Complication are due to production of exotoxin	• Caused by *Corynebacterium diphtheriae* • Droplet infection and can infect skin lesion	• Greyish membrane in throat • Clinical picture

Clinical features	Treatment	Prevention

• Catarrh for about $\frac{2}{52}$
• Cold, lasting $\frac{3}{52}$ - $\frac{4}{52}$
• Cough
  — chronic
  — paroxysmal
  — may lead to bleeding in
    in eyes and eyelids
• Whoop, this is uncommon in
  child under $\frac{6}{12}$ age
• Vomiting after whoop
• Apnoeic and/or cyanotic
  attacks in a baby under $\frac{3}{12}$
• Complications
  — pneumonia
  — malnutrition
  — convulsions
  — otitis media
  — encephalitis
  — hernia
	• 50 mg/kg **Chloramphenicol**
	  in catarrhal stage
	• **Penicillin** or **Ampicillin** for
	  complications
	• Feed after vomiting
	• Sedation at night with
	  Promethazine (but observe
	  carefully)
	• ?oxygen therapy ⎱ may or may
	• ?humidification ⎰ not help
	• Artifical ventilation for
	  apnoea, if available
		• Vaccinate

• Begins as a mild illness
  — child tires easily and is
    lethargic
  — anorexia
  — neck swollen slightly
  — whitish membrane in
    throat
  — moderate fever
• Acute illness (at 4-6 days)
  — neck very swollen
  — greyish membrane in
    throat (necrotic tissue,
    WBC exudate and
    bacteria)
• Complications:
  — tracheal obstruction
  — heart failure due to
    myocarditis (at 10–14
    days)
  — spreads to nerves and
    child unable to swallow or
    breathe (at 3–7 weeks)
  — septicaemia
	• Give **Penicillin** and
	  Antitoxin (10 000–100 000)
	  unit IV/IM) immediately,
	  after test dose
	• Give oxygen if available
	• Steroids may ↓ oedema
	• Humidification may help
	• Tracheostomy and suction
	  PRN
	• Observe heart rate, pulse,
	  colour and respiratory rate
	• Keep in hospital for at least
	  $\frac{2}{52}$ to make sure that
	  myocarditis is not developing
	• Treat complications PRN,
	  NG tube feeding may be
	  necessary
	• The patient should rest
		• Vaccinate

Disease and incubation period	General notes	Pathology and aetiology	Diagnosis
Polio 5-30 days, usually 10 days	• Associated with poor hygiene; but if there is no immunisation, and ↑ in hygiene will → ↑ paralytic polio, as later age of onset • In developing countries, most children infected by 4 years. Peak incidence in 2nd year • Incidence of paralytic polio is 1%, but ↓ risk if child young	• Viral infection; there are 3 strains • Transmitted by droplet and faeco-orally	• Clinical picture *but* majority of children with polio will have no symptoms at all
Tetanus 6-15 days	• Some passive immunity at birth therefore vaccinate all pregnant women	• Caused by *Clostridium tetani* • Infection through open wound, however small • Complications result from the toxin which is produced	• Clinical picture

Clinical features	Treatment	Prevention

Days 1-3
• Child unwell with symptoms of 'flu
• Fever
• Person may appear to recover
 	
Days 3-5
• Headache ⎱ due to viral
• Stiff neck ⎰ meningitis
• Fever
• Pains in muscles
 	
Days 5-7
• Mild paralysis
 	
or
• Severe paralysis
  — asymmetrical
  — affects legs more than arms
  — affects large muscle groups
  — no sensory loss
	• Rest paralysed limbs in position where contractures will not develop
	• Passive and active movements of limbs (i.e. physiotherapy)
	• Refer to orthopaedic consultant if paralysis permanent, for calipers etc.
	
	Paralysis will not get any worse after 2 weeks following onset of the disease but improvement may take 1-2 years
		• Vaccinate
		• Improve hygiene

In newborns: • Tight mouth • Baby stops sucking • Spasm and stiffness of the body • Fits *In older children and adults:* • 'Risus sardonicus' (mouth tight and twitching) • Opisthotonus • Stiffness of muscles • Spasm of muscles in response to sound — painful • Malaise • Fever and sweating • Headache • Irritability • Dysphagia ⎱ due to spasm of • Asphyxia ⎰ larynx and respiratory muscles	• Debride wound • Give antibiotics • Give 5 000 units human tetanus immunoglobulin (HTIG) *or* Give 10 000 units antitetanus serum IV (750 units to baby) • Give adults 8 mg/day **Betamethasone** • Sedate and relax muscles with 0.2 mg/kg **Valium** PO or IM *or* 1 mg/kg **Promethazine** syrup via NG tube *or* 0.1–0.2 ml/kg/dose **Paraldehyde** • If tachycardia > 120/min, give **Propranolol** • Keep noise, unnecessary movement and injections etc. to a minimum • Maintain hydration and electrolyte balance, feed via NG tube • Physiotherapy • Heparin to prevent DVT if unconscious • General nursing care	• Immunise *all* children and adults • Give pregnant mothers tetanus toxoid ×2, one month apart • Wash hands and use sterile equipment to cut (and dress) umbilical cord • Careful hygiene of cord postnatally

Vaccination

Vaccine	Type	Storage			
		Refrigerator (not freezer)		Room temperature	
		Undiluted	Diluted	Undiluted	Diluted
DPT *'Triple'*	Diphtheria–toxoid Pertussis–dead bacteria Tetanus–toxoid	2–8°C Do *not* freeze	2–8°C 2–3 years		2–3 days
		(If liquid clear 5 min after shaking it, it is useless)			
Measles	Live attenuated freeze-dried vaccine	Up to 8°C May be frozen $\frac{6}{12}$	7–8 hours	Away from sunlight 1–2 days	5–6 hours
Polio (Sabin)	Live attenuated virus, containing 3 strains	−15°C − −25°C May be frozen	6 months		2 days
BCG	Live attenuated freeze-dried bacteria	4–8°C Away from sunlight 1–2 years	2–3 hours	1 month in cold room	1–2 hours
Tetanus	Toxoid	4–8°C Do *not* freeze	2–3 years		2–3 days
Cholera	Dead bacteria	4–8°C Do *not* freeze 2 years	6–8 hours	1–2 days	1 hour
Yellow fever	Live attenuated virus, freeze-dried	May be frozen 1 year	1 hour	1–2 days	1 hour
Monovalent Typhoid	Dead bacteria		Do not freeze 2 years		2 days
Rabies (Merieux)		4°C			

Administration	Dose	Contra-indication	Age	Reactions
SC or IM injection in thigh 3 injections at least $\frac{1}{12}$ apart	Usually 0.5 ml	High fever	1st $\frac{2}{12} - \frac{3}{12}$ 2nd $\frac{2}{12} - \frac{3}{12}$ later 3rd $\frac{2}{12} - \frac{3}{12}$ later School entry (DT only)	Fever 12–24 hours later Pain at injection site for 24 hours
IM injection in thigh × 1	Usually 0.5 ml	Treat TB and malnutrition first if possible	$\frac{6}{12}$ –3 years $\sim \frac{9}{12}$ recommended	Mild fever and slight rash at 6–10 days
Oral × 3 at least one month apart	3 drops	Diarrhoea or vomiting	1st $\frac{2}{12} - \frac{3}{12}$ 2nd $\frac{2}{12} - \frac{3}{12}$ later 3rd $\frac{2}{12} - \frac{3}{12}$ later	None
Intradermal injection on ® shoulder × 1	Varies with make of vaccine 0.05 ml often	Known TB	Birth to 12 years	Lymphadenitis
SC or IM injection × 3 for primary course, then one booster if pregnant again or injury	Usually 0.5 ml	None	Any age or antenatal	Pain at injection site for 12–24 hours
SC injection × 2, 1–2 wks apart for 1° course One booster every $\frac{4}{12} - \frac{6}{12}$	1–10 yrs 0.5 ml Over 10 yrs 1 ml	Acute illness, chronic heart, liver or kidney disease	1 year to any age	Pain at injection site for 24 hours
SC injection × 1 Lasts for 10 years	Usually 0.5 ml	Under 1 year, acute illness, 1st trimester of pregnancy	1 year to any age	Mild fever, malaise for 24 hours
Deep SC injection × 2 at interval of $\frac{6}{52}$. Booster × 1 every $\frac{12}{12}$	Varies	Acute infection, TB, heart or kidney disease	1 year to any age	Pain at injection site and mild fever for 48 hours
0.1 ml on day 0 28 and $\frac{6}{12}$. Lasts 3 years. SC injection				

Malnutrition

A child's nutritional status will significantly affect:
- Physical development
- Motor development
- Intellectual development

Therefore assessment of nutritional status and correction of nutritional deficiency is *vital*.

Promotion of adequate growth

'The promotion of adequate growth is a more positive objective than prevention of malnutrition'

(Morley)

1 **Good antenatal care** (see *THCN Obstetrics*)
- Promote maternal health in pregancy
- Prevent intra-uterine growth retardation
- Prevent premature delivery

2 **Encourage breast-feeding**

3 **Ensure balanced diet before and after weaning**
- Start introducing other foods apart from breast milk at 4–6 months
- Give gruel and mashed fruit first
- Give food after breast-feed
- Introduce one new food at a time
- Gradually increase amounts
- Children need to be fed 4–6 times per day up to 3 years of age (may need change in family eating habits)
- Continue breast-feeding for as long as possible
- Use 'Food Square' to plan balanced meals that are not too bulky for a child to eat—one item from each square per meal

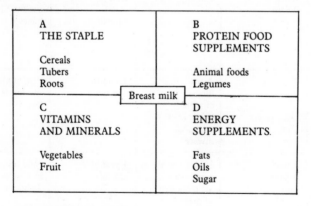

4 **Do *not* stop feeding sick children**

5 **Protect from infectious disease and treat parasitic disease**

6 **Encourage growth of nutritionally valuable crops**
- Train in agricultural methods
  - fencing/terracing
  - soil preparation
  - composting
  - hillside water conservation etc.
- Educate as to what is nutritionally valuable to grow

7 Identify those at risk of malnutrition

Assess nutritional status
- Increase in WEIGHT
  - compare this with 'reference' weights of children of the same age
  - chart weight on 'Road to Health' chart
  - it is the direction in which a child's weight curve is going which is important
- Arm circumference (e.g. Shakir strip, Echeverri tape)
  - increases in the first year, then remains fairly constant from 1–5 years therefore *single* AC measurements more useful than *single* weight

Whatever **'Road to Health'** chart is used, it must:
  - be home based
  - include insert for medical problems and treatment
  - include social history
  - 'At Risk' register to be kept

THE ARM CIRCUMFERENCE

(1) Use a tape measure. Measure the child's left arm. Let it hang by his side with his elbow straight. Measure his arm circumference half way between the point of his shoulder and his elbow.

Put the tape gently, but firmly, round his arm. Don't pull so tight that folds come in his skin.

(2) You can also measure a child's arm circumference with a 1 cm strip of old X-ray film.

Soak the film in hot soda for a day. Wash off the 'picture' with hot water. Make a scratch down the film at 0 cm. Make two more scratches at 12·5 cm and 14 cm. Colour the film below 12·5 cm red with a spirit pen. Colour the film yellow between 12·5 and 14 cm. Colour it green above 14 cm. Put the red colour close to the scratches, but don't let it touch them. Cut the film into 1 cm strips.

A child with an arm circumference below 12·5 cm is severely malnourished. If his arm circumference is between 12·5 cm and 14 cm, he is moderately malnourished. If it is above 14 cm, he is normal.

You can also use a piece of coloured string to measure the arm circumference. It is not so good because it stretches.

The arm circumference is NOT helpful in children under one year or over five years.

A CHILD WITH AN ARM CIRCUMFERENCE OF LESS THAN 14 CM BETWEEN THE AGES OF ONE AND FIVE IS MALNOURISHED

---

tape

green = normal

yellow = moderate malnutrition

red = severe malnutrition

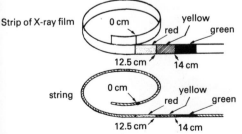

Measuring the arm circumference

Identify those at risk of malnutrition (continued)

- Keep an **'At Risk'** register; the following factors are associated with an increased risk of malnutrition (Morley et al, 1979)
  - birth weight below 10th percentile - ♂ 2.4 kg, ♀ 2.3 kg
  - failure to gain 0.5 kg/month in 1st 3 months of life or 0.25 kg/month in 2nd 3 months of life
  - twins or other multiple births
  - all birth orders over 7
  - short birth intervals
  - maternal weight < 43.5 kg (96 lb)
  - breakdown of marriage or death of either parent
  - more than four sibling deaths
  - breast infections and difficulties in breast-feeding, particularly those secondary to maternal psychiatric illness
  - an episode of measles, whooping cough and severe repeated diarrhoea in the early months of life
  - physical or mental handicap in child
  - recent migration of mother to the area

Provide a home-based record for these children and keep a copy yourself. Make them a priority for home visits.

- Combine **Antenatal** and **Child Health** clinics, providing curative and preventive care. If care is available for mother and child at the same time, you will get better attendance and coverage of the population.

Nutritional deficiency disease	Clinical features
Kwashiorkor 'moon' face sparse, weak, red or grey hair anaemia noticeable in conjunctivae 'flaking paint' rash apathetic features 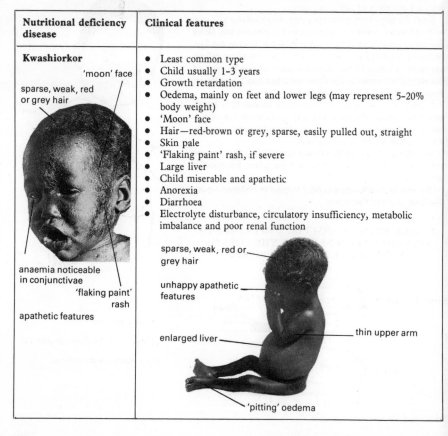	• Least common type • Child usually 1–3 years • Growth retardation • Oedema, mainly on feet and lower legs (may represent 5–20% body weight) • 'Moon' face • Hair—red-brown or grey, sparse, easily pulled out, straight • Skin pale • 'Flaking paint' rash, if severe • Large liver • Child miserable and apathetic • Anorexia • Diarrhoea • Electrolyte disturbance, circulatory insufficiency, metabolic imbalance and poor renal function sparse, weak, red or grey hair unhappy apathetic features enlarged liver thin upper arm 'pitting' oedema

Nutritional deficiency disease	Clinical features
Marasmus 'little old man' features hair normal— 'potbellied' little subcutaneous fat and gross muscle wasting grossly underweight	• Most common type • Often in children < 1 year • Short and light for age • Shrunken and wizened as no subcutaneous fat • Marked muscle wasting • Usually hungry • No oedema • Prone to measles and *Herpes simplex*
Vitamin A deficiency (Xerophthalmia)	• Night blindness • Photophobia • Conjunctiva dry and slightly rough • Bitot's spots (foamy whitish-grey patches) at side of eye • Corneal cloudiness • Corneal ulceration and scarring • Keratomalacia — cornea opaque and soft; rapid destruction of eyeball, cornea bursts → **blindness**
Vitamin D deficiency (Rickets)	Caused by lack of exposure to sunlight • Misshapen bones, including pelvis • Enlarged bones at wrist and ankles
Anaemia (see page 19)	• Pallor of lips, tongue, conjunctiva and hands • Shortness of breath • Tired and listless • Rapid pulse • Swollen feet
Vitamin C deficiency (Scurvy)	Vit C is needed for absorption of iron • Anorexia • Poor wound healing • Anaemia
Vitamin B deficiency • Thiamine (B_1) ('Beri-beri') • Niacin ('Pellagra') • Riboflavin (B_2)	 • Red, sore tongue • Weakness • Anorexia • Swelling of ankles and feet • Peeling sores or dry, cracked skin where exposed to sun • Cracking, soreness and dryness of lips, corners of mouth and in the angles of the nose

Definition of malnutrition

Weight as % of standard (i.e. 50th percentile · Harvard values)	Oedema	
	Present	Absent
60–80%	Kwashiorkor	Underweight
< 60%	Marasmic-kwashiorkor	Marasmus

Aetiology of malnutrition

- Undernutrition
  It used to be thought that marasmus was a protein and calorie deficiency, and that kwashiorkor was just protein deficiency, but it is *now* thought that a calorie deficiency is the main problem. Food given to children is often too bulky for them to eat enough to provide the necessary calories.
- Infection, with associated anorexia (especially measles)
- Aflatoxin (Professor Hendrickse's work)
  ↑ levels of **aflatoxin** (i.e. aspergillus mould affecting peanuts and legumes) in urine of children with kwashiorkor and marasmus, but higher in kwashiorkor. It is therefore possible that both malnutrition *and* fungal toxins are needed for kwashiorkor to develop, *or* possibly those with kwashiorkor are unable to metabolise aflatoxin → hypoproteinaemia.

Treatment of malnutrition

Mild and moderate malnutrition

NB *Involve parents* in *ALL* care and give nutritional education
- Improve diet (including advice to mothers re right foods etc.)
- Feed more frequently
- Give supplementary foods PRN, but avoid making family dependent on this
- Monitor child's weight and health regularly

Severe malnutrition

Should be treated in hospital or health centre:
For last 3–4 days **Resuscitation**: 20–40% will die during this stage unless handled properly
From 5 days **Rehabilitation**

1. Take history
   - Breast-feeding/time of weaning/what eaten in last 24 hours
   - When last smiled
   - Recent disease/contact with TB
2. Examine patient
   - Send MSU to screen for infection
   - Look for signs of xerophthalmia
   - Look for signs of other infections and infestations such as malaria, hookworm, TB
3. Give suppressive dose of **Chloroquine** on admission as a routine if malaria is a common problem in the area
4. Give IM injection 100 000 IU water-miscible **Vitamin A** on admission (or 200 000 IU orally) and repeat orally on 2nd day. Give 50 000 IU to child under 1 year.
5. If Hb < 3 g/100 ml, give blood transfusion
6. Correct dehydration, if necessary, and maintain hydration
7. Prevent hypoglycaemia (common cause of death)
   - Feed frequently
   - If blood glucose < 1 mmol/l, give extra **Glucose**. May also give 0.5 mg/kg **Prednisone** 6 hrly to mobilise glycogen stores.
   - If consciousness reduced, give IV **Glucose**

8 Protect from hypothermia — i.e. temp $< 35.6°C$ (96°F)
- Don't wash child in 1st 4 days
- Nurse away from open windows
- Keep well clothed and covered, especially at night
- Get mother to carry child around with her (constant source of heat)

9 Give vitamin and mineral supplements
- 1 g **Potassium chloride** daily
- **Iron**
- 5 mg **Folic acid** daily
- **Multivitamins** (Vit B_1, B_2, niacin, Vit A, Vit D, Vit C, Vit B)

10 Prevent heart failure (severe and often fatal complication, especially in Kwashiorkor)
- Observe for signs of ↑ respiratory rate, hepatomegaly, triple rhythm, ↑ oedema, ↓ Hb
- Use low sodium diet
- ? use **Frusemide (Lasix)** to get rid of oedema

11 Start dietary treatment as soon as child no longer dehydrated (see below)

To make full strength milk feeds, using what milk is available locally

	Cow's milk	Whole milk powder	Dried skimmed milk	K-mix Z (UNICEF)	Yoghourt
Milk	1000 ml	150 g	75 g	100 g	1000 ml
Sugar	50 g	50 g	50 g	—	50 g
Oil	20 g	10 g	60 g	70 g	20 g
Water (boiled and cooled)	—	Make up to 1000 ml	Make up to 1000 ml	Make up to 1000 ml	—
		(mix other ingredients to paste with some of water, then add the rest of the water)		—	—

Typical feeding schedule for severely malnourished child (with above feed)

Days in centre	Type of feed	Daily dosage	Divided into
1	Half-strength milk feeds	150 ml/kg body weight	12 feeds/day
2	Half-strength milk feeds	150 ml/kg body weight	8 feeds/day
3 and 4	$\frac{2}{3}$ strength milk feeds	150 ml/kg body weight	8 feeds/day
5 onwards	Full-strength milk feeds	150 ml/kg body weight	6 feeds/day

- After 1st 7-10 days when dehydration and infections cleared and the child takes oral feeds well, increase feeds to 200 ml/kg/day to allow for catch-up growth
- Can use nasogastric tube at first, then wean on to oral feeds
- If diarrhoea occurs, dried skimmed milk could be exchanged for casein

Health education

Health education is a vital part of any patient's care. Whenever a patient is seen, there is an opportunity for teaching and this must be taken if we are to:
- Help people help themselves
- Prevent disease
- Contribute to the quality of life
- Avoid the consequences of unrecognised and/or neglected illness

Health education may be given:
a) **On an individual basis**
    i.e. while examining and treating a patient
b) **On a group basis**
    i.e. for both inpatients and outpatients
c) **On a community basis**
    i.e. in the village or town or school situation

Teaching needs to be:
- Prepared well
- Enthusiastically carried out
- Simply taught
- Enhanced with good visual aids
- Made relevant to the local situation and local resources
- Evaluated as to its effectiveness, and adjusted as necessary

Prevention is still better than cure

A very useful reference in this field is:
Werner, D. and Bower, B. (1982) *Helping Health Workers Learn,* (available from TALC)

Health education, in whatever context, should involve consideration of the following general areas:

Promotion of good health

1   Good balanced diet (see pages 88–93)
2   Immunisation (see pages 86–87)
3   Hygiene
    - Personal
    - Food   } (see pages 96–97)
    - Household
    - Community
4   Home safety

Management of simple health problems

1   Diarrhoea and oral rehydration
2   Coughs and colds
3   Management of fever
4   First aid
5   When to seek medical advice

Parentcraft

1 Pregnancy
   - Coming for antenatal care
   - What problems to report
2 Labour
   - What to expect
   - How the mother can help herself
3 Puerperium
   - Recovery from delivery
4 Baby
   - Feeding
   - General baby care
   - Introduction to 'Road to Health' chart and child health clinics
5 Parenting skills
   - Promoting general health of the child
   - Promoting development of the child
   - Coping with problems
6 Family planning

Basic hygiene

Personal hygiene

- Bathe often, every day if possible (to prevent skin infections etc.)
- Wash hands with soap and water after having a bowel movement and before eating
- Wear shoes (to prevent hookworm infection)
- Brush teeth daily using toothbrush and toothpaste (if no toothbrush make one by fraying the end of a twig, and use mixture of salt and bicarbonate of soda as toothpaste)

Food hygiene

- If possible, boil all drinking water; once boiled, protect by putting in a container with a lid
- Do not let flies crawl on food; protect food by keeping it covered or in a wire mesh cupboard
- Wash fruit and vegetables before eating raw if they have been on the ground
- Cook all meat and poultry thoroughly

Household hygiene

- Teach all members of the family, including children, to use a latrine (see diagram of latrine, page 97)
- Wash cups, plates etc. well and put out in the sun to dry on a clean surface above ground level (this surface can be made with a few sticks — see diagram)
- Hang sheets and blankets in the sun often to air them; if bedbugs are a problem, wash linen on the same day and pour boiling water on the cots/beds
- Do not spit on the floor as this can spread disease
- Clean house often and fill in cracks in the walls etc.
- Try to keep animals outside the house
- Delouse the family frequently, if fleas or head/body lice are a problem; treat all the family at the same time

Community hygiene

- Try to prevent the spread of infection by getting sick people to sleep separately from other well people
- Encourage the use of latrines and discourage urination and defaecation into rivers or onto the ground
- Protect the water supply (see diagram of protected well, page 97)
- Treat all diseases promptly
- Ensure that children and pregnant women receive all the necessary vaccinations
- If refuse can be burned, burn it, otherwise bury it in special place or use for compost (see diagram of composting)

Composting

Use of organic refuse (i.e. not tins, metal, plastic) to provide low-cost fertiliser

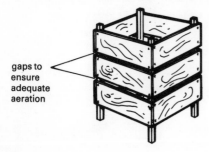

gaps to ensure adequate aeration

- Make about 1 metre square with wood *or* poles and wiremesh
- For each 9 in (23 cm) refuse, put 2 in (5 cm) soil on top, then 9 in refuse, then 2 in soil etc.
- Make sure it is well aerated

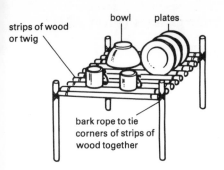

Drying stand for cups, plates, dishes etc.

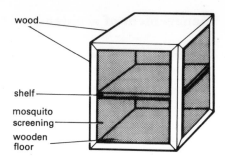

Wire mesh cupboard to protect food

Improved pit latrine

- Line the top of the pit to prevent collapse
- Vent pipe: flies are drawn up the pipe to the light if the inside of the latrine is dark; there is a fly trap at the top
- Paint the inside of latrine dark
- Site the latrine downhill from any water source, if possible (if above well, site to one side)
- Concrete squat plate — may be covered

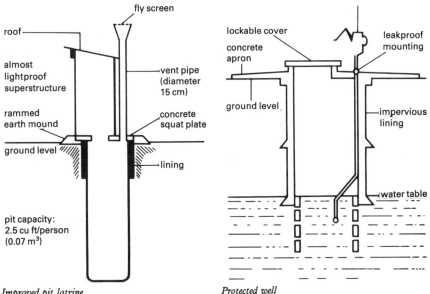

Improved pit latrine   *Protected well*

Protected well

The following are needed to construct the well
- Impervious lining for a minimum of 3 m (more if gravel or sand)
- Concrete apron around the well, sloping away from the well mouth
- Extend the lining to provide a headwall—the top of the wall should be narrow to prevent people standing on it
- Fence area around to exclude animals from the well
- Lid or cover for well top

Restrict the use of private buckets if there is no pump
Site at least 15 m away from a latrine (30 m if gravel, more if limestone)

Management of accidents and emergencies (First Aid)

The *priorities* in any situation are:
Airway   — clear
Breathing — adequate
Circulation — cardiac function
               — arrest any bleeding
               — hydration
This applies *both when treatment is initiated and as it continues*. Any other measures are, in comparison, secondary.

Cardiac arrest

- Clear airway of vomit, dislodged teeth etc., *quickly*
- Have the patient on a firm surface
- Perform external cardiac massage   *and* ● Mouth-to-mouth resuscitation
- adult: 60/min using whole hands (heel)   — head slightly extended
  on sternum   — make firm seal with mouth over mouth
- child: 60–100/min — less pressure used   — pinch nose
  than for adult   — give 1 breath for every 4 pumps of cardiac
- baby: 100–140/min — use two fingers only   massage
- check carotid pulse to ensure that massage is   — make sure lungs are inflating with each breath
  effective
- When respiration and circulation are restored: observe patient closely for further problems (in hospital)
- Try to ascertain and correct cause of cardiac arrest

If the patient's heart has stopped for more than 3 minutes, irreversible brain damage is likely to have occurred.

Choking

A child

- Turn the child upside down and slap him/her on the back

An adult

- Stand behind the patient and put your arms round his/her waist, placing your fist between the ribs and the umbilicus of the patient
- Press into the patient's abdomen with your fist with a sudden strong upward jerk. Repeat as necessary to dislodge the foreign body.

A patient who is already unconscious

- Lie him/her on back
- Sit over patient with heel of hands over one another (as in cardiac massage) between ribs and umbilicus
- Give quick, strong, upward push
- Repeat as necessary
If the treatment has not been successful, try mouth–to–mouth resuscitation.

Drowning

A child

- Try to turn the child upside down quickly and get the water out of the lungs
- Start mouth-to-mouth resuscitation and cardiac massage as necessary

An adult

- Try to drain out any water that comes out easily — do not take long doing this
- Start mouth-to-mouth resuscitation and cardiac massage as necessary
If the patient recovers, place him/her in the 'recovery' position and observe closely in hospital

Bleeding

- Raise the injured part higher than the rest of body, if possible
- Place a clean cloth on the wound and press *hard*. Keep pressing until bleeding stops (may be 15-60 min). If the cloth gets soaked, do not remove it but place another clean cloth on top of it and maintain the pressure.
- If bleeding + + + and pressure does not help, apply a tourniquet but you *must* release for a few seconds every 20 min to avoid gangrene. Transfer to hospital.
- When the bleeding has stopped, dress the wound and replace the lost fluid and blood

Shock

Causes

- Blood loss
- Extensive burns
- Dehydration
- Extreme pain
- Severe illness
- Anaphylactic reaction (allergy)

Signs

- BP < $\frac{90}{60}$
- Pulse rapid and weak
- Cool clammy skin
- ↓ consciousness
- Weakness
- Mental confusion

Treatment

- Lie the patient in the 'recovery' position with the head lower than rest of the body
- Ensure adequate breathing and circulation
- Stop any bleeding (see previous section)
- Replace fluid as quickly as possible via intravenous infusion — use **Hartmann's solution** (Ringer's lactate) if available
- Monitor pulse, blood pressure and general condition carefully
- Give pain relief, if the patient is in great pain
- Reassure the patient, if he/she is conscious
- If the patient is not in hospital, transfer him/her to hospital

Loss of consciousness

- Place in 'recovery' position (i.e. on side with face down so that, if any vomiting, there is less risk of inhalation)

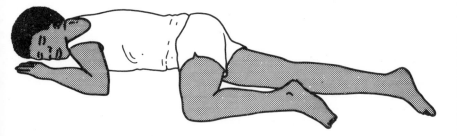

Recovery position

- Give fluids (and food) by IVI or NG tube, until consciousness has fully returned
- Turn 2 hrly to avoid development of pressure sores
- Monitor fluid input and output; there will probably be a need to catheterise the patient
- Observe the pulse, BP, respirations, level of consciousness, size and reaction of pupils half hrly
- If cardiac or respiratory arrest occurs, give cardiac massage and/or mouth-to mouth resuscitation (if only respiratory arrest, just give mouth-to mouth resuscitation)
- Investigate and treat cause

Fever

- Remove the patient's clothing
- If his/her temperature ≥ 40°C in an adult or ≥ 38°C in a child, start tepid sponging i.e. wet cloths in lukewarm water (*not* cold) and place on the patient, replace as they warm and dry with more wet cloths
- Give **Aspirin** or **Paracetamol** to ↓ fever
- Treat any infection or malaria or other cause
- Be aware of the risk of febrile convulsion in a child
- Teach the patient and a relative how to manage fever (for future use)

Burns

Prevention

Prevention is *much* better than cure
- Protect children from fires of all kinds
- Lock away all liquids that could burn

Treatment

- Immediately (or as soon as possible) place the burnt area under cold running water or immerse it in cold water for 10 min
- Cover the burn with a clean, dry cloth until medical help is obtained
- Assess the degree of the burn:
  - 1° **redness only** ⎫ It may be difficult to decide whether the burn is 2°
  - 2° **blistering of skin** ⎬ or 3° at first, but in 3° the skin will eventually
  - 3° **blistering and skin destruction** ⎭ turn grey. Treatment is the same at first.
- Clean the burn with cooled boiled water with antiseptic added
- Dress with **Vaseline** gauze (if no commercial gauze available, sterilise Vaseline by heating and cooling, then applying it to the sterile gauze); *never* use other grease or butter if no Vaseline gauze is available, leave it uncovered and dust it with **Antibiotic powder**
- If the burn is severe, it may induce shock, so give extra fluids PO or IV; if alert and conscious, give ORS (see page 55); if ↓ consciousness and unable to drink frequently, use IVI of normal **saline** or, preferably, **Hartmann's solution**
- Give pain relief
- If large burn, give prophylactic **Antibiotics**
- Change dressings as necessary, using *sterile* technique
- Avoid contractures — put **Vaseline** gauze between two burnt surfaces (e.g. fingers) to avoid them healing stuck together; encourage movement; 3° and some 2° burns will need skin grafting

Cuts and wounds

Background

Need to know:
- How long it is since the injury occurred
- Is the wound clean or contaminated
- Is there other damage e.g. fractures, damage to internal organs or blood vessels
- Was wound cause by an animal bite, if so, there is the danger of rabies and tetanus

Treatment

- Clean with **antiseptic** solution. If it is a big wound, pour in **Hydrogen peroxide** or **Potassium permanganate** solution or cooled boiled water and clean the wound with a *sterilised* nail brush. Whatever the size of the wound, make sure it is *really clean*. Remove all foreign bodies.
- Cut away any damaged skin or tissues (debridement), preserving important blood vessels and nerves. If there is bleeding, put a hot pack on it to stop the bleeding. Tie off any bleeding vessels. (Damaged fat is grey rather than yellow; damaged muscle is not bright red and does not contract.)

- *If it is a small wound, with no contamination, little damage, and it is less than 8 hours since injury:*
  - butterfly suture (if shallow)

Butterfly suture

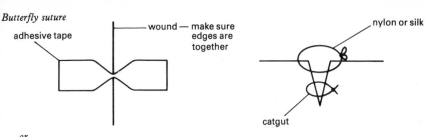

or
  - suture each layer individually with nylon or silk to skin, and catgut to underlying tissues

Types of sutures

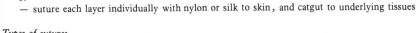

continuous   interrupted (use reef knot)   mattress

  - do not create a dead space i.e. the depths of the wound must be sutured in layers

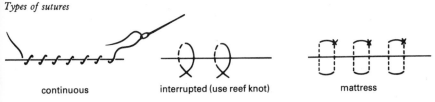

  - do not tie muscle sutures too tightly as will cause necrosis
  - make sure skin edges are aligned and not inverted

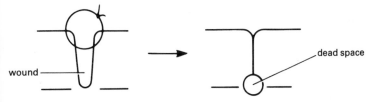

- *If*
  - *> 8 hours since injury and/or*
  - *contamination of wound and/or*   } Do *NOT*
  - *damage to tissue and other structures*   suture
                                               immediately
  Infection is much more likely in this situation therefore:
  - clean
  - debride
  - dress
  - observe for signs of infection
  - give **Antibiotics** if infection or high risk of infection

  After 3-7 days:
  - assess wound again
  - debride again, as necessary
  - if the wound is clean and there are no signs of infection stitch the wound
  - continue observation of the wound for infection and treat accordingly

Fractures

This is a specialised subject and only the principles will be outlined here. A useful reference book is Sir John Charnley's *The Closed Treatment of Common Fractures* (Churchill Livingstone).

Aims of treatment

- To reduce fracture
- To maintain bone in correct position
- To immobilise while healing takes place

Treatment

- Do *not* force when trying to reduce fractures
- Do *not* put a plaster cast over an open wound
- An X-ray is needed to make sure the fracture is reduced correctly
- If there is a possibility of fracture of the spine, keep the patient immobilised while transferring him/her to hospital and keep him/her immobilised afterwards

Snake bites

(with acknowledgements to Dr. Alistair Reid's lecture notes)
- Reassure patient
- Wipe site of bite (do *NOT* incise)
- If, and only if, large amount of venom has been injected, tie a crepe bandage firmly above site of bite (not too tightly) and transfer the patient to hospital
- If venom from a spitting cobra enters the eyes, bathe the eyes promptly and repeatedly in water (if no water is available, use saliva or even urine)
- If the patient is vomiting, place him/her in the recovery position
- Move the bitten limb as little as possible
- Observe pulse, BP, respiratory rate and condition of site of bite
- *ONLY* give antivenom if
  — local swelling present
  — bite of necrotising snake (e.g. cobra, puff adder) and < 4 hours after injury
  — systemic signs (palsy, abnormal bleeding, myalgia, shock, cardiac or respiratory problems)
  Watch out for signs of anaphylactic shock due to venom

Index

milk feeds, 93
molluscum contagiosum, 46–7
mosquito, 16

ORS, 55
oedema, 23
onchocerciasis, 38–9, 40–1, 46, 62–3
Opisthorchis spp., 60–1
oriental sore, 74–5

Paragonimus spp., 60–1
paralysis, 85
parentcraft, 95
pellagra, 46–7, 91
phlyctenular conjunctivitis, 36–7
pig tapeworm, 58–9
pit latrine, 97
pityriasis, 44–5
plasma, 12–13
pneumonia, 24–5
polio, 84–5, 86–7
pregnancy, 19, 29
pterygium, 40–1
pulse, 22
pupil reaction, 31
pyoderma, 42–43

rabies, 78–9, 86–7
rehydration, 55
relapsing fever, 46, 67, 76–7
remedies, simple, 7
renal tract, TB of, 28
resources, 6
respiration, 23
respiratory disease, 8, 23–7
rheumatic fever, 24–5
rickets, 91
rickettsiosis, 76–7

ringworm, 44–5
river blindness; *see* onchocerciasis
rotavirus, 52–3
roundworm, 56–7

SI units, 13
Sabin vaccine, 86–7
Salmonella spp., 50–1
sandfly, 74
scabies, 9, 44–5
schistosomiasis, 8, 19, 52–3, 64–5
scrub typhus, 34
scurvy, 91
serum, 12–13
sexually transmitted disease, 68–71
shock, 30, 99
sickle-cell disease, 19, 20, 67
skin conditions, 9; allergic, 46–7; bacterial, 42-5; due to deficiency, 46–7; fungal, 44–5; parasitic, 44–5; TB of, 29; viral, 46–7
sleeping sickness, 72–3
snake bites, 102
spleen, enlarged, 20
squint (strabismus), 40–1
stress, and sickling, 20
Strongyloides spp., 56–7
stye, 40–1
'swimmers' itch', 65
syphilis, 42–3, 68–9

tapeworms, 58–9
tetanus, 34–5, 84–5, 86–7
Tetrapetalonema sp., 62–3
thalassaemia, 19, 21
threadworm, 58–9

thrush, 44–5
thyrotoxicosis, 40
ticks, 9, 76
Tinea versicolor, 44–5
Toxicara canis, 58–9
trachoma, 9, 38–9
Trichinella spp., 58–9
Trichomonas vaginalis, 70–1
Trichuris, 52–3
trypanosomiasis, 34, 46, 72–3
trypsin inhibitor, 50
tuberculoid leprosy, 48
tuberculosis, 8, 28–9, 36–7
tumbu fly abcess, 44–5
typhoid, 9, 44–5, 86–7
typhus, 46, 76; scrub, 34

ulcers, 42–3
urethritis, non-specific, 70–1
urine, normal values, 12–3

vaccination, 86–7
vitamin deficiency: A, 38–9, 91; B, 46–7, 91; C, 19, 91; D, 91

water, 96, 97
weaning, 52–3
well, protected, 97
whipworm, 52–3, 56–7
whole blood, 12–13
whooping cough, 82–3
worms, 8, 56–63
wounds, 100–1
Wuchereria bancrofti, 62–3

xerophthalmia, 38–9, 91

yellow fever, 66, 86–7